PROGRESS IN CLINICAL AND BIOLOGICAL RESEARCH

RECENT TITLES

Vol 79: **Proteins in the Nervous System: Structure and Function,** Bernard Haber, Jose Regino Perez-Polo, Joe Dan Coulter, *Editors*

Vol 80: **Mechanism and Control of Ciliary Movement,** Charles J. Brokaw, Pedro Verdugo, *Editors*

Vol 81: **Physiology and Biology of Horseshoe Crabs: Studies on Normal and Environmentally Stressed Animals,** Joseph Bonaventura, Celia Bonaventura, Shirley Tesh, *Editors*

Vol 82: **Clinical, Structural, and Biochemical Advances in Hereditary Eye Disorders,** Donna L. Daentl, *Editor*

Vol 83: **Issues in Cancer Screening and Communications,** Curtis Mettlin, Gerald P. Murphy, *Editors*

Vol 84: **Progress in Dermatoglyphic Research,** Christos S. Bartsocas, *Editor*

Vol 85: **Embryonic Development,** Max M. Burger, Rudolf Weber, *Editors.* Published in 2 volumes: Part A: **Genetic Aspects** Part B: **Cellular Aspects**

Vol 86: **The Interaction of Acoustical and Electromagnetic Fields With Biological Systems,** Shiro Takashima, Elliot Postow, *Editors*

Vol 87: **Physiopathology of Hypophysial Disturbances and Diseases of Reproduction,** Alejandro De Nicola, Jorge Blaquier, Roberto J. Soto, *Editors*

Vol 88: **Cytapheresis and Plasma Exchange: Clinical Indications,** W.R. Vogler, *Editor*

Vol 89: **Interaction of Platelets and Tumor Cells,** G.A. Jamieson, *Editor;* Alice R. Scipio, *Assistant Editor*

Vol 90: **Beta-Carbolines and Tetrahydroisoquinolines,** Floyd Bloom, Jack Barchas, Merton Sandler, Earl Usdin, *Organizers*

Vol 91: **Membranes in Growth and Development,** Joseph F. Hoffman, Gerhard H. Giebisch, Liana Bolis, *Editors*

Vol 92: **The Pineal and Its Hormones,** Russel J. Reiter, *Editor*

Vol 93: **Endotoxins and Their Detection With the Limulus Amebocyte Lysate Test,** Stanley W. Watson, Jack Levin, Thomas J. Novitsky, *Editors*

Vol 94: **Animal Models of Inherited Metabolic Diseases,** Robert J. Desnick, Donald F. Patterson, Dante G. Scarpelli, *Editors*

Vol 95: **Gaucher Disease: A Century of Delineation and Research,** Robert J. Desnick, Shimon Gatt, Gregory A. Grabowski, *Editors*

Vol 96: **Mechanisms of Speciation,** Claudio Barigozzi, *Editor*

Vol 97: **Membranes and Genetic Disease,** John R. Sheppard, V. Elving Anderson, John W. Eaton, *Editors*

Vol 98: **Advances in the Pathophysiology, Diagnosis, and Treatment of Sickle Cell Disease,** Roland B. Scott, *Editor*

Vol 99: **Osteosarcoma: New Trends in Diagnosis and Treatment,** Alexander Katznelson, Jacobo Nerubay, *Editors*

Vol 100: **Renal Tumors: Proceedings of the First International Symposium on Kidney Tumors,** René Küss, Gerald P. Murphy, Saad Khoury, James P. Karr, *Editors*

Vol 101: **Factors and Mechanisms Influencing Bone Growth,** Andrew D. Dixon, Bernard G. Sarnat, *Editors*

Vol 102: **Cell Function and Differentiation,** G. Akoyunoglou, A.E. Evangelopoulos, J. Georgatsos, G. Palaiologos, A. Trakatellis, C.P. Tsiganos, *Editors.* Published in 3 volumes. Part A: **Erythroid Differentiation, Hormone-Gene Interaction, Glycoconjugates, Liposomes, Cell Growth, and Cell-Cell Interaction.** Part B: **Biogenesis of En-**

ergy Transducing Membranes and Membrane and Protein Energetics. Part C: **Enzyme Structure—Mechanism, Metabolic Regulations, and Phosphorylation-Dephosphorylation Processes**

Vol 103: **Human Genetics,** Batsheva Bonné-Tamir, *Editor,* Tirza Cohen, Richard M. Goodman, *Associate Editors.* Published in 2 volumes. Part A: **The Unfolding Genome.** Part B: **Medical Aspects**

Vol 104: **Skeletal Dysplasias,** C.J. Papadatos, C.S. Bartsocas, *Editors*

Vol 105: **Polyomaviruses and Human Neurological Disease,** John L. Sever, David Madden, *Editors*

Vol 106: **Therapeutic Apheresis and Plasma Perfusion,** Richard S.A. Tindall, *Editor*

Vol 107: **Biomedical Thermology,** Michel Gautherie, Ernest Albert, *Editors*

Vol 108: **Massive Transfusion in Surgery and Trauma,** John A. Collins, Kris Murawski, A. William Shafer, *Editors*

Vol 109: **Mutagens in Our Environment,** Marja Sorsa, Harri Vainio, *Editors*

Vol 110: **Limb Development and Regeneration.** Published in 2 volumes. **Part A,** John F. Fallon, Arnold I. Caplan, *Editors.* **Part B,** Robert O. Kelley, Paul F. Goetinck, Jeffrey A. MacCabe, *Editors*

Vol 111: **Molecular and Cellular Aspects of Shock and Trauma,** Allan M. Lefer, William Schumer, *Editors*

Vol 112: **Recent Advances in Fertility Research,** Thomas G. Muldoon, Virendra B. Mahesh, Bautista Pérez-Ballester, *Editors.* Published in two volumes. Part A: **Developments in Reproductive Endocrinology.** Part B: **Developments in the Management of Reproductive Disorders**

Vol 113: **The S-Potential,** Boris D. Drujan, Miguel Laufer, *Editors*

Vol 114: **Enzymology of Carbonyl Metabolism: Aldehyde Dehydrogenase and Aldo/Keto Reductase,** Henry Weiner, Bendicht Wermuth, *Editors*

Vol 115: **Prevention of Hereditary Large Bowel Cancer,** John R.F. Ingall, Anthony J. Mastromarino, *Editors*

Vol 116: **New Concepts in Thyroid Disease,** Roberto J. Soto, Gerardo Sartorio, Ismael de Forteza, *Editors*

See pages following the index for previous titles in this series.

NEW CONCEPTS IN THYROID DISEASE

NEW CONCEPTS IN THYROID DISEASE

Proceedings of the International Symposium Held in Buenos Aires, Argentina, October 6–8, 1981

Editors

Roberto J. Soto
Gerardo Sartorio
Ismael de Forteza

Fundación Argentina de Endocrinología
Buenos Aires, Argentina

Alan R. Liss, Inc., New York

Address all Inquiries to the Publisher
Alan R. Liss, Inc., 150 Fifth Avenue, New York, NY 10011

Library of Congress Cataloging in Publication Data

International Symposium on "New Concepts in Thyroid
Disease" (1981: Buenos Aires, Argentina)
New concepts in thyroid disease.

(Progress in clinical and biological research; v. 116)
Bibliography: p.
Includes index.
1. Thyroid gland—Diseases—Congresses. I. Soto,
Roberto J. II. Sartorio, Gerardo. III. Forteza,
Ismael de. IV. Fundación Argentina de Endocrinología.
V. Title. VI. Series. [DNLM: 1. Thyroid diseases—
Congresses. W1 PR668E v.116/WK 200 I58 1981]
RC655.I64 1983 616.4′4 82–24926
ISBN 0-8451-0116-1

FAE FUNDACION ARGENTINA DE ENDOCRINOLOGIA

Contents

Contributors

Syed M. Amir [207]
Beth Israel Hospital and Harvard Medical School, Boston, Massachusetts 02215

Marta Barontini [105]
Centro de Investigaciones Endocrinológicas, Hospital de Niños Ricardo Gutierrez, Gallo 1330, 1425 Buenos Aires, Argentina

Rubén José Boado [105, 131]
Endocrine Research Laboratory (PLABIEN), CONICET, Center of Nuclear Medicine, Hospital de Clínicas José de San Martín, Córdoba 2351, 1120 Buenos Aires, Argentina

D.P. Cardinali [105]
Centro de Estudios Farmacológicos y de Principios Naturales (CEFAPRIN), Serrano 665/669, 1414 Buenos Aires, Argentina

G. D. Chazenbalk [57]
División Bioquímica Nuclear, Comisión Nacional de Energía Atómica, Avda. del Libertador 8250, 1429 Buenos Aires, Argentina

Ana María Cortizo [57]
Centro de Endocrinología Experimental y Aplicada (CENEXA), Instituto de Embriología, Biología e Histología, Facultad de Ciencias Médicas, Universidad Nacional de La Plata, Calles 60 y 120, 1900 La Plata, Argentina

Leslie J. DeGroot [1]
Department of Medicine, University of Chicago, 950 East 59th Street, Chicago, Illinois 60637

T. De Paoli [45]
Depto. de Físico Matemáticas, Facultad de Farmacia y Bioquímica, Universidad de Buenos Aires, Junín 956, 1113 Buenos Aires, Argentina

J. J. Gagliardino [57]
Centro de Endocrinología Experimental y Aplicada (CENEXA), Instituto de Embriología, Biología e Histología, Facultad de Ciencias Médicas, Universidad Nacional de La Plata, Calles 60 y 120, 1900 La Plata, Argentina

C. L. Gómez Dumm [57]
Centro de Endocrinología Experimental y Aplicada (CENEXA), Instituto de Embriología, Biología e Histología, Facultad de Ciencias Médicas, Universidad Nacional de La Plata, Calles 60 y 120, 1900 La Plata, Argentina

A. A. Hager [45]
Depto. de Físico Matemáticas, Facultad de Farmacia y Bioquímica, Universidad de Buenos Aires, Junín 956, 1113 Buenos Aires, Argentina

Sidney H. Ingbar [207]
Beth Israel Hospital and Harvard Medical School, Boston, Massachusetts 02215

G. J. Juvenal [105]
Comisión Nacional de Energía Atómica, Avda. del Libertador 8250, 1429 Buenos Aires, Argentina

The boldface number in brackets following each contributor's name indicates the opening page of that contributor's paper.

Robert D. Leeper [139]
Nuclear Medicine Service, Memorial Hospital, 1275 York Avenue, New York, NY 10021

Geraldo Medeiros-Neto [119, 155]
Thyroid Laboratory, Hospital das Clinicas, Faculdade de Medicina da Universidade de São Paulo, C. Postal 8091, 01000 São Paulo, Brasil

P. I. Oteiza [45]
Depto. de Química Biológica, Facultad de Farmacia y Bioquímica, Universidad de Buenos Aires, Junín 956, 1113 Buenos Aires, Argentina

J. M. Pasquini [45]
Depto. de Química Biológica, Facultad de Farmacia y Bioquímica, Universidad de Buenos Aires, Junín 956, 1113 Buenos Aires, Argentina

M. A. Pisarev [57, 105]
Comisión Nacional de Energía Atómica, Avda. del Libertador 8250, 1429 Buenos Aires, Argentina

Koshi Saito [169, 189]
Department of Endocrinology and Metabolism, Jichi Medical School, Minamikawachi, Tochigi, Japan

J. Enrique Silva [23, 75]
Peter Bent Brigham Hospital, Thyroid Unit, 721 Huntington Avenue, Boston, Massachusetts 02115

E. F. Soto [45]
Depto. de Química Biológica, Facultad de Farmacia y Bioquímica, Universidad de Buenos Aires, Junín 956, 1113 Buenos Aires, Argentina

V. Sridama [1]
Department of Medicine, University of Chicago, 950 East 59th Street, Chicago, Illinois 60637

Takaji Takai [169, 189]
Department of Endocrinology and Metabolism, Jichi Medical School, Minamikawachi, Tochigi, Japan

Edgardo Ulloa [131]
Endocrine Research Laboratory (PLABIEN), CONICET, Center of Nuclear Medicine, Hospital de Clínicas José de San Martín, Córdoba 2351, 1120 Buenos Aires, Argentina

M. I. Vacas [105]
Centro de Estudios Farmacológicos y de Principios Naturales (CEFAPRIN), Serrano 665/669, 1414 Buenos Aires, Argentina

Kunihiro Yamamoto [169, 189]
Department of Endocrinology and Metabolism, Jichi Medical School, Minamikawachi, Tochigi, Japan

Sho Yoshida [169, 189]
Department of Endocrinology and Metabolism, Jichi Medical School, Minamikawachi, Tochigi, Japan

Angel A. Zaninovich [131]
Endocrine Research Laboratory (PLABIEN), CONICET, Center of Nuclear Medicine, Hospital de Clínicas José de San Martín, Córdoba 2351, 1120 Buenos Aires, Argentina

Preface

Intensive basic and clinical research in endocrinology has resulted in a rising flow of information which must be absorbed by the practitioner. This need for constantly updating applicable knowledge extends, of course, to thyroidology as well. Second only to diabetes as the most frequent endocrine disease, disturbances of the thyroid are understood much better today due to the combinative efforts of researchers in immunology, cell biology, and molecular biology. It is with the intention of advancing this base of knowledge in as coherent and concise a manner as possible that we publish these proceedings.

In the following pages we present the work of some of the outstanding scientists who contributed to the International Symposium on New Concepts in Thyroid Disease, held in Buenos Aires, October 6–8, 1981. This was the fifth meeting sponsored by the Fundación Argentina de Endocrinología (FAE) in the last three years and displays the FAE's goal of linking basic and clinical research together in an effort to enhance progress in the field of endocrinology.

We wish to thank the publishers and the participants in the meeting for their willingness to help the FAE in achieving this goal.

Roberto J. Soto
Gerardo Sartorio
Ismael de Forteza

New Concepts in Thyroid Disease, pages 1–22

DEVELOPMENT OF THYROID AUTOIMMUNITY

Leslie DeGroot
V. Sridama
Thyroid Study Unit, Department of Medicine,
The University of Chicago,
Chicago, Illinois, U.S.A.

In the two and a half decades since first recognition of thyroid autoantibodies by Doniach and Roitt, (1956) and Rose and Witebsky (1956), we have learned a great deal about general concepts of autimmunity and their pathogenetic role in autoimmune thyroid diseases. In Graves' disease, Hashimoto's thyroiditis, and idiopathic myxedema, which are closely related diseases, circulating antibodies are formed against thyroglobulin (Doniach, D., 1957), other colloid antigens (Doniach, D., 1975), microsomal proteins (Mariotti, S., 1979), and components of TSH receptors (Adams, D.D., 1967 - Fenzi, G., 1979). The central role of TSH receptor antibodies in producing thyrotoxicosis (Clague, R., 1976 - O'Donnell, J., 1978) has been documented. Cell-mediated immunity,which recognize thyroid antigens (Lamki, L., 1973 - Aoki, N.,1979) and orbital tissue antigens (Kalman, K.,1978) have been demonstrated in Graves' and Hashimoto's patients. T-lymphocytes appeared to play a prominent role in this process (Okita, N.,1980). Circulating immune complexes containing thyroid antigens have been recognized (Mariotti, S., 1979 - Ohtaki, S., 1981). Deposits of immune complexes (Kalderon, A.E., 1977) and immunoglobulins (Werner, S.C., 1972) in thyroid tissues and extraocular muscle membranes (Konishi, J., 1974) also occurred. Patients with thyroid autoimmunity often develop autoimmunity against other organs (Friedman, I., 1978 - Doniach, D., 1979), including adrenal cortex, parathyroid gland, gastric parietal cells, gonads, pancreatic islets, and occasionally the pituitary gland, and sometimes have associated non-organ specific autoimmunity of the collagen-vascular variety (Doniach, G., 1975). While the occurrence, distribution, and pathogenic significance of these immune reactions has been extensively studied, causal factors have not been identified.

Pre-Graves' Disease

It is interesting (and possibly important) to recognize the early stages of autoimmune thyroid diseases and to observe the evolution of such immunological and thyroid functional abnormalities in predisposed population, since it is well documented that hereditary factors are pathogenetically involved in Graves' disease (Friedman, I, 1978). Offspring of parents who have had Graves' disease are an ideal population for such studies. Therefore, we have undertaken a longitudinal study of children of parents who have Graves' disease, and a control population selected from volunteers who have no known first degree relatives with thyroid disease. Our initial report provided data on 153 children of parents with Graves' disease and 129 control children. The evaluation consisted of history, physical examination, and a variety of thyroid function and immunological tests. Any alteration in size or consistency of the thyroid gland, presence of exophthalmos or vitiligo, or deviation from from normal in serum assays for thyroxine, free thyroxine index, triiodothyronine, TSH, thyroglobulin, thyroglobulin hemagglutinating antibodies, and microsomal hemagglutinating antibodies were classified as an abnormality.

TABLE 1
Percentage of Graves' disease children or controls with abnormalities

	Controls				Graves'Disease Children			
Age Group	6-15	16-25	26->30	6->30	6-15	15-25	26->30	6->30
Female	9.1	38.2	15.4	24.6	31.8	38.7	42.8	36
Male	15.4	10.9	29.4	23.3	31.4	38.9	36.4	34.4
Total	11.4	31.2	23.3	24.0	31.6	40.8	40.0	35.5

TABLE 2
Percentage distribution of total abnormalities of Graves' disease children (GDC) and controls (CC).

	Thyroid	FTI	TGHA	MCHA	TSH	T3	Vitiligo	Thyro-toxicosis
GDC	13.1	3.3	11.1	7.8	2.6	9.1	1.3	2
CC	6.9	2.3	9.3	7.8	0.8	6.2	0	0

Thirty-six percent of children of Graves' patients had one or more abnormalities, as compared to 24% of the control group (Table 1) (De Groot, L., 1980). It was of great interest that the types of abnormalities found in Graves' children and controls were similar in variety and intensity, and differed primarily in frequency (Table 2). There is obviously room in such a study for considerable bias on the part of the examiner, who frequently knew which group the children belonged in. However, half of the thyroid abnormalities detected by physical examination were accompanied by laboratories' abnormalities such as high or low thyroid hormone level, abnormal thyroglobulin, or the presence of antithyroid antibodies. One quarter of all children having minor abnormalities in the thyroid gland might be diagnosed as having Hashimoto' thyroiditis on the basis of small goiter and postive antibodies. There was a dramatic clustering of abnormalities in certain families. Thirteen families had two or more abnormal children per family, whereas 21 families had no abnormal children. A bioassay for Long Acting Thyroid Stimulator, using the McKenzie technique (McKenzie, J., 1967), was infrequently positive -- of 2 of 95 children of Graves' patients, and 1 of 49 control children. Thyropin displacing immunoglobulins measured by radioreceptor assay (Fenzi, G., 1979) were uniformly negative. Assays for cell-mediated immunity against thyroid particulate antigens and thyroglobulin, using a blastogenesis assay (Aoki, N., 1979), were also uniformly negative.

It was of special interest to follow this group of children during subsequent years, whether there were detectable abnormalities or not at the time of the first visit. We examined 59 members of the original cohort of Graves' disease children one or more years later. Among 24 of these who originally had an abnormality, 13 had lost it, 13 retained it, and 8 had acquired a new abnormality. Among 35 children who originally had no detectable abnormality, 9 later acquired an abnormality. In many children, progressive development of autoimmunity has been documented, including individuals who gradually developed goiter and elevated free thyroxine index with mild clinical hyperthyroidism, who developed exophthalmos or vitiligo or a progressive increment in thyroid antibody levels and evidence of hipothyroidism. The child who developed mild clinical and chemical hyperthyroidism responded to three months of antithyroid drug therapy with a prolonged remission in thyrotoxicosis.

These studies document a surprisingly high prevalence of minor thyroid abnormalities in allegedly normal children, and are similar to the observation of Tunbridge (1977), in Wickham, England. Among our normal control children there was at least a 4% incidence of Hashimoto' thyroiditis. It was striking that Hashimoto' thyroiditis was found in both the control and children of Graves' patient population, but the 3 cases of Graves' disease found, were present only among the children of parents with this anomaly. Among children of parents with Graves' disease, thyroid abnormalities are more common than in controls. The abnormalities increase in incidence with age, and are not stable. Some abnormalities subsequently disappear, and others appear. The immunological abnormality in these children is a dynamic evolving state. Sometimes there is a propensity for autoimmunity to worsen, and at other times control factors within the individual apparently suppress the abnormality. It is our hypothesis that such waxing and waning of autoimmunity leads in time to the full blown clinical state of Graves' disease. Furthermore, we suggest that, if such abnormalities can be detected at a very early stage of clinical development, it may be possible to reverse the development through the use of antithyroid medication or other treatments.

Previous studies in relatives of Graves' patients also showed several thyroid abnormalities, including an increased incidence of thyroid autoantibodies (Roitt, I., 1967), abnormal TRH tests (Chopra, I., 1977 - Tamai, H., 1980), increased incidence of cell- mediated immunity against thyroid particulate antigen (Farid, N., 1974). One follow-up study (Tamai, H., 1980) showed some individuals who were found to be TRH-hyporesponders, who later developed clinical hyperthyroidism and several cases of abnormal TRH response which normalized during the follow-up period.

Histocompatibility antigens may play a role in familial aggregation of Graves' disease, since it has been well documented that HLA B_8 antigen (Whittingham, S., 1975) (Grumet, F., 1974 - Ford, D., 1976) and more striking, HLA-Dr_3 (Beck, K., 1977 - Farid, N., 1979), are associated with Graves' disease in Caucasian populations, and possibly HLA-Dr_5 (Weissel, M., 1980 - Farid, N., 1981) with Hashimoto's thyroiditis (goitrous type). We are currently evaluating the HLA antigens of our cohort of Graves' disease children and may subsequently be able to correlate the familial aggregation and development of thyroid abnormalities with the presence of these antigens.

The Role of Immune Complexes

Thyroglobulin is a ubiquitous serum antigen, and patients with autoimmune thyroid disease commonly develop antithyroglobulin antibodies. Thus the stage is set for the formation of immune complexes, and theoretically for the development of immune complex disease. It is interesting that immune complex disease has in fact rarely been encountered in clinical thyroid autoimmunity, there being a total of about five cases in which pathologically important renal deposits of thyroglobulin containing immune complexes have been reported (O'Regan, S., 1976 - Ploth, D., 1978 - Horvath, F., 1979 - Jordan, S., 1978 - Jordan, S., 1981).

We studied nonspecific circulating immune complexes using a Raji cell RIA method and found elevated values in 3 of 18 patients with Hashimoto' thyroiditis, 4 of 39 with thyroid carcinoma, and none of 21 with Graves' disease (Mariotti, S., 1979). Thyroglobulin could not be found in the immune conplexes bound to Raji cells when sought by a sensitive antibody technique. Further, we found that, when human antithyroglobulin was mixed with human thyroglobulin, the complexes formed did not bind complement and did not attach to Raji cells. In contrast, when human thyroglobulin was mixed with rabbit antithyroblobulin antibody, the complexes did fix complement and bind to Raji cells. Thus, human antithyroglobulin and its antigen form complexes which poorly fix complement (Mariotti, S., 1979). This may be a fortunate characteristic of such immune complexes, allowing them to be cleared from the circulation and not form tissue deposits, especially in the kidney, which cause immune complex disease.

Specific thyroglobulin containing immune complexes were assayed in these patients using the Kriss method (Takeda, Y., 1977). Low levels of thyroglobulin containing immune complexes were detected in 5% of patients with thyroiditis, 38% of patients with Graves' disease, and 33% of patients with thyroid cancer (Fig. 1). There was no correlation between the nonspecific immune complex levels and the specific thyroglobulin containing immune complex levels.

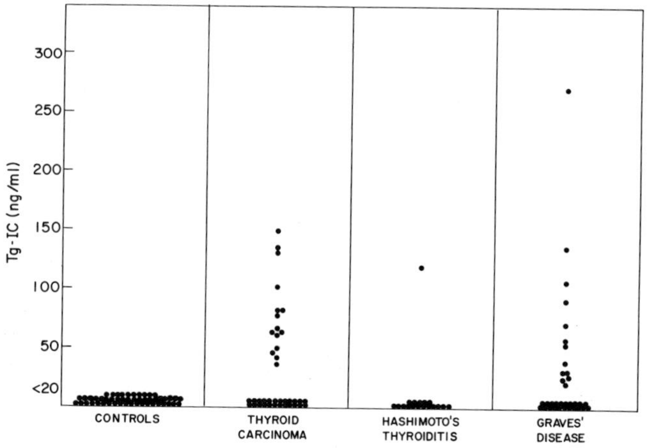

Fig. 1.- Levels of circulating Tg-ICs by radioassay in 50 normal controls and 90 patients with thyroid disease (Mariotti, S., 1979).

The dynamic formation of these immune complexes was demonstrated by Mariotti et al (1980) in studies conducted on patients after trauma to the thyroid gland from thyroid surgery or needle aspiration cytology. These procedures stimulated the release of thyroglobulin into the circulation, followed by formation of immune complexes in patients who had circulating antithyroglobulin antibody, and then a marked reduction in circulating antibody titers. Over a period of one to two days, the immune complexes were cleared, thyroglobulin disappeared, and the suppressed antithyroglobulin antibody level returned to its previous level (Fig. 2). Thus immune complexes are formed in these circumstances and are rapidly cleared from the circulation, usually without tissue damage. It is known that antithyroglobulin antibody levels are lower and less prevalent in patients with Graves' disease than in Hashimoto's thyroiditis. Possibly this is because thyroglobulin is constantly released from the hyperstimulated Graves' disease thyroid, forms immune complexes with circulating antithyroglobulin antibody, which are continuously cleared from the circulation, causing a suppression of serum antithyroglobulin antibody titers.

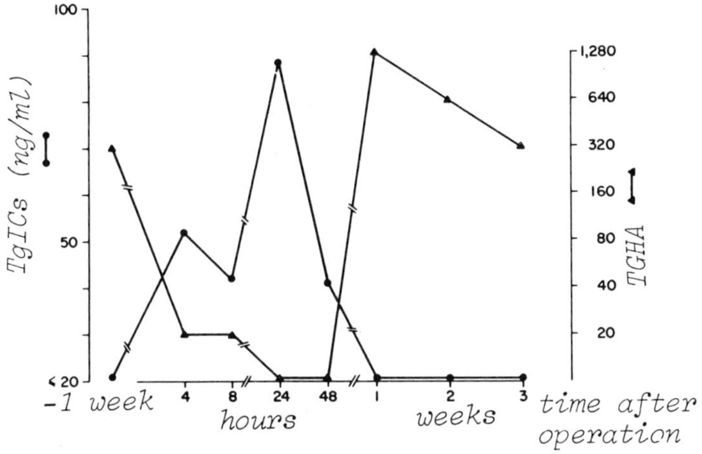

Fig. 2.- Levels of anti-Tg antibody TGHA, ▲-----▲) and Tg-anti-Tg immune complexes (TgICs ●-----●) in a patient with Graves' disease one week before and at different time intervals after subtotal thyroidectomy (Mariotti, S., 1980).

Thus, thyroglobulin and antithyroglobulin immune complexes occur in human autoimmune thyroid diseases, but their overall pathogenic significance is uncertain. Because of their failure to fix complement, they do not commonly cause immune complex disease. However, it is possible that the formation of immune complexes on the surface of the thyroid cell may be a factor leading to the thyroid cell death typical of Hashimoto's thyroiditis and idiopathic myxedema.

Suppressor Cell Studies in Graves' Disease

Many factors in the natural history of autoimmune thyroid disease, perhaps most strikingly the dynamic changes seen in the Graves' disease children, suggest that there may be an abnormality in the control mechanisms in the immune system. Suppressor cells, which modulate the ability of other cells to mount an immune reaction, are one such factor. Suppressor functions are present in several types of cell, including monocytes, and especially T lymphocytes which act on helper T cells or directly inhibit immunoglobulin synthesis by B cells (Waldmann, T., 1978). Abnormalities in suppressor cell function have been detected in several autoimmune diseases, such as SLE (Bresnhian, B., 1977 1977 - Sakane, T., 1978), rheumatoid arthritis (Chattopadhyay, C., 1979), and multiple sclerosis (Antel, J., 1978 - Gonzalez R., 1979), and correlate with the activity of such diseases.

We have inverstigated suppressor cell function in patients qith Graves' disease and Hashimoto' thyroiditis using assays of Concanavalin-A induced suppressor cell activity and short lived suppressor cell function (Aoki, N., 1979). We found that suppressor cell activity was deficient in patients with active Graves' disease, and returned toward normal as patients improved with therapy (Fig. 3). More recently we measured immunoglobulin synthesis in re - constituted mixtures of T and B cells of Graves' patients (Pacini, F., 1981). When B cells were incubated alone *in vitro*, immunoglobulin synthesis was low. Upon addition of T cells, immunoglobulin production was increased, probably due to a helper effect. Using lymphocytes from normal subjects, when the ratio of T to B cells was gradually increased, suppression of immunoglobulin synthesis eventually occurred. In Graves' patients there was no inhibition of immunoglobulin synthesis, even with high ratios of T to B cells, indicating a suppressor cell deficit (Fig. 4). Graves' B lymphocytes responded normally to suppression by T lymphocytes from normal subjects, but not if the normal T cell population had been treated by radiation to destroy the suppressor cells. Radiation did not alter the result when T lymphocytes from Graves' patients were used. Thus, again, there was evidence for a deficient function of suppressor cells in patients with active Graves' disease.

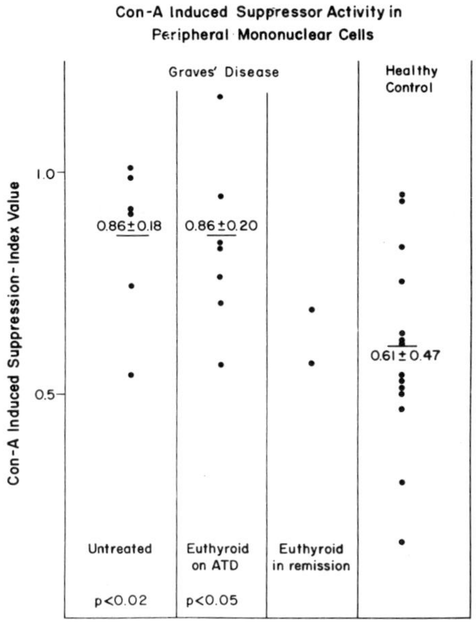

Fig. 3.- Con A-induced suppressor activity in the patients with Graves' disease and in healthy subjects. ATD, Antithyroid drugs. (Aoki, N., 1971)

This defect has been confirmed by enumeration of subsets of T lymphocytes using monoclonal antibodies directed against specific cell surface antigen of T cells. The percentage of suppressor cells, as defined by reaction with the OK-T_8 antibody in peripheral mononuclear cells, was reduced in toxic untreated Graves' disease, but improved and normalized after treatment (Fig. 5) (Sridama, V., 1981).

While diminished function and number of nonspecific suppressor cells has been documented in patients with Graves' disease, it is uncertain whether this is a primary or secondary abnormality. It is possible that the deficiency represents the functional loss of suppressor cells due to the production of anti-lymphocyte antibodies, or a change in function of suppressor cells which have been activated by

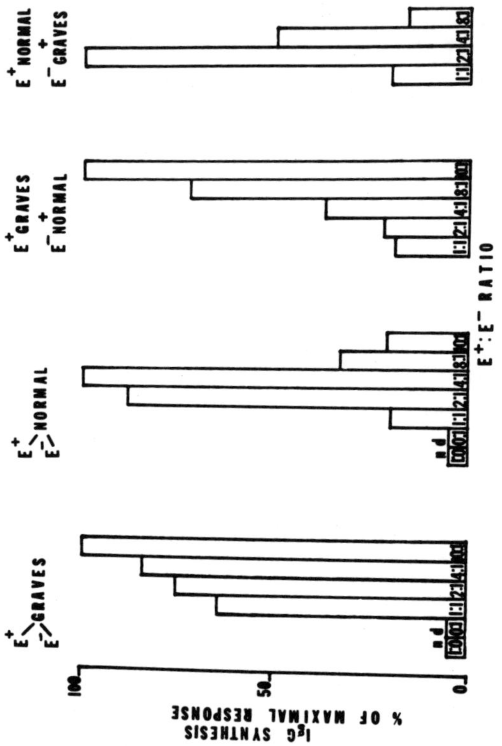

Fig. 4.- IgG synthesis by B cells (0.2 x 10^6/tube) co-cultured with increasing numbers of T cells. Representative experiment using syngenic and allogeneic combinations of cells from one normal control and one patient. Data are expressed as % of maximal response. nd = not detectable (Pacini, F., 1981)

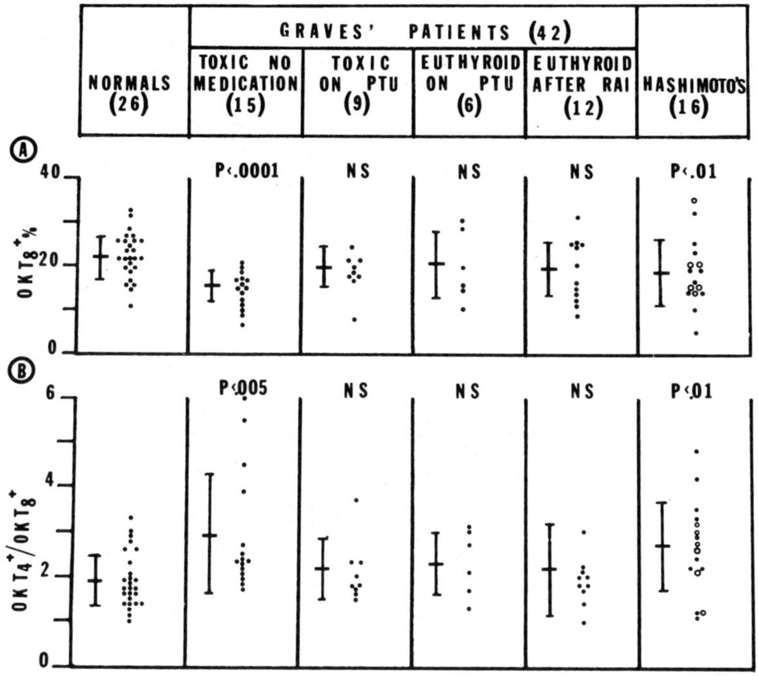

Fig. 5.- Percentage of OK T_8^+ cells (A) and OK T_4^+ / OK T_8^+ ratio (B) in patients with Graves' disease, Hashimoto's thyroiditis, and normal controls. °Indicates patients without hormone treatment in the Hashimoto's group. The brackets represent the mean $\pm$ std. dev. # indicates subjects per group (Sridama, V., 1981)

circulating immune complexes. It is also possible that such suppressor cells are low in the blood because they move into peripheral tissues. It will be very important to document specific suppressor cell activity using a plaque forming assay specific for thyroglobulin antibody producing cells. Such plaque forming assays have now been developed in a number of laboratories, including those of McLachan, S., (1981) and Davies, T., (1981). Specific thyroglobulin producing plaque forming cells can be quantitated and have been shown to be increased in the circulation of patients with Graves' disease and thyroiditis.

Possible Mechanisms of Thyroid Auto-immunity

The mechanism of thyroid auto-immunity remains uncertain and many hypotheses have been proposed (Fig. 6).

We can consider these in relation to anti-thyroglobulin antibody production.

In the normal individual TG is present at low levels in the circulation and is believed to provide "low dose suppression" of T lymphocytes, so that they do not provide, the "help" required by B lymphocytes present in the circulation, and able to produce antibody.

Thus, minimal amounts of anti-TG Ab are produced.

Greatly increased exposure to TG may overcome this suppression.

We found half of thyroid cancer patients examined to have a blastogenic response to TG (Aoki, N., 1979) and this correlated with high serum TG levels.

Viral or other damage to thyroid cells could lead to an altered TG molecule to which T cells could responde, providing help to B cells.

This could lead, as in experimental thyroiditis (Weigle, W., 1969) to production of antibody to the abnormal antigen, and this antibody could cross- react partially with normal TG.

Possibly maternal antibody could cross the placenta and eliminate fetal TG from the circulation, thus preventing the fetal "self-recognition" process and allowing T lymphocytes after birth to help B cells to make antibodies.

This could not explain paternal transmission of the disease.

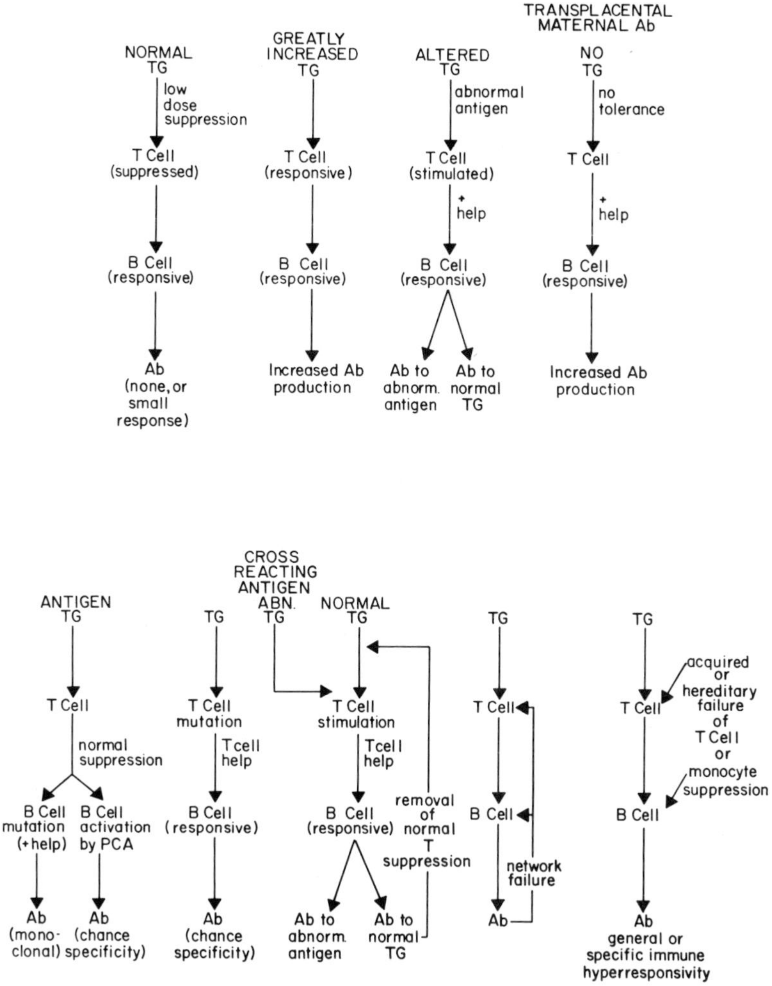

Fig. 6.- Hypotheses offered to explain development of antithyroglobulin antibodies. See text for details.

Volpé has proposed (Lamki, L., 1973 - Okita, N., 1980) that mutational changes could be responsible for chance production of auto-immunity.

Mutated T lymphocytes (a process not generally

recognized) would provide specific Th help or detection of specific Ts cells. Theoretically B cell mutation (Burnet, F., 1959) could produce chance monoclonal anti-TG antibodies as in myeloma. The clear HLA associations, the gradual temporal progression of the illness, the multiplicity of thyroid (and other organ) antibodies and CMI responses involved, and the apparent ability of the process to return from an abnormal to quasi-normal state in some circumstances all suggest that a mutational theory is too simplistic.

An extension of the altered antigen theory has been proposed, in which the cross-reacting antibody removes antigen from the circulation and this eliminates normal low dose T lymphocyte suppression (Weigle, W., 1969).

Ig is known to control its own synthesis by feedback mechanisms.

One process involves formation of anti-idiotype antibodies. These prevent action of or suppress production of the first antibody. This "Idiotype network" may regulate B and perhaps T cell functions. Dysfunction of the network would allow unchecked Ab synthesis.

Anti-idiotype Ab have not so far been recognized in auto-immune thyroid disease, but probably exist.

Much current speculation revolts around demonstrations of reduced suppressor cell function (Waldmann, T., 1978).

These suppressor cells (possibly monocytes, specific Ts cells or subsets of the Th cells) may have generalized suppressor function or may be antigen specific. A decrease in suppressor cell function has been proposed as a pathogenic feature of multiple sclerosis (Antel, J., 1978 - Gonzalez, R., 1979) rheumathoid arthritis (Chattopadhyay, C., 1979), lupus (Bresnhian, B., 1977 - Sakane, T., 1978), myastenia gravis and by us in auto-immune thyroid disease (Aoki, N., 1979 -Sridama, V., 1981). Possibly both, generalized and antigen specific suppressor cell abnormalities will be found. We doubt that an isoloated defect in Ts controlling one type of antibody will be the cause of auto-immune thyroid disease, because of the multiplicity of antigens involved, and because the immune system seems to function with many interlocking types of checks and balances. However, the clear demonstrations of reduced suppressor cell numbers and function in Graves' disease and thyroiditis indicate that they probably play a role in the development of the process and in the "vicious cycle" positive feedback induced by the thyrotoxic state. Altered Th/Ts ratios also probably explain in part the amelioration of thyrotoxicosis in pregnancy and the frequent post-partum exacerbations.

At this time we hypothesize that auto-immune thyroid disease, Graves', Hashimoto's, and Gull's are extremely closely linked variants of some fundamental immune pathology. A satisfactory explanation for their pathogenesis must explain the widespread occurrence of auto-antibodies, the genetic predisposition, the fluctuating nature of the illnesses,the impact of stress on the illness (if any), and the final outcome hypothyroidism. No contemporary theory provides this holistic concept. As a working, fragmentary model we offer the following sequence.

1.- Auto-immunity to thyroid antigens-thyroglobulin and "microsomal" is present normally in most people at very low levels and can be detected by current tests in at least 12-16%.

2.- Genetic factors including inheritance of specific MHL antigens B8, Dw3 and Dw5 certain Gm immunoglobulin allotypes and abnormal suppressor cell function predisposes some of the population to augmented antibody formation and cell mediated immune responses.

3.- Stress acting via increased TG (and other antigen) release and via adrenal stimulation may alter the balance of T lymphocyte help, or Ts/Th ratio, in favor of increased immunity.

4.- Antibodies and cell mediated immunity (steps 1-3) damage the thyroid releasing antigens and expanding the antigenic repertoire with increased antibody titers and formation of new antibodies such as thyroid stimulating and thyrotrophin displacing antibody and eye tissue reactive antibodies.

5.- Thyroid stimulating antibodies cause Graves thyrotoxicosis if the thyroid can respond. Thyrotoxicosis itself has a positive feedback on the process by augmenting immune reactivity, perhaps by several mechanisms, one of which is reduced Ts cells.

6.- Antibodies and CMI gradually destroy the thyroid producing the clinical pictures of goitrous thyroiditis and primary thyroid failure.

7.- During the early phase of the process the balance between expansion or suppression of the immune response depends upon function of idiotype feedback and suppressor cells. These may (especifically if Graves thyrotoxicosis is controlled) be enough to either prevent progressive clonal expansion or bring the disease to a clinically inactive state although the immune diathesis persists.

8.- Progressive cell damage leads in time to thyroid failure.

Abstract

In thyroid autoimmune diseases, including Graves' disease, Hashimoto's thyroiditis, and idiopathic myxedema, patients develop antibodies against thyroglobulin, microsomal protein, and TSH receptors, cell-mediated immunity against thyroid antigens, circulating immune complexes, and tissue deposition of immune complexes. Other organ-specific autoimmunity often co-exists. The basic abnormality has not been identified.

To recognize the early phase of autoimmunity, we studied thyroid and serological abnormalities in children of parents with Graves' disease, and found that 36% had some detectable thyroid related abnormality compared to 24% of a control group. The physical or chemical abnormalities presaged the development of thyrotoxicosis in some patients, often were associated with clinical thyroiditis, changed from year to year, and were specifically prevalent in some families These studies emphasize the inheritance of thyroid disfunction, and the instability of the lesion during its early development.

Immune complexes were studied by nonspecific complement dependent assays (C1Q and Raji cell systems), and were found in 3 of 18 patients with thyroiditis and none of 21 with Graves' disease. Thyroglobulin immune complexes were not identified by these techniques, but could be detected using the Kriss radiometric assay. Thyroglobulin containing immune complexes were present in 5% of patients with thyroiditis and 38% of patients with Graves' disease. Thyroid damage was found in some patients to cause release of thyroglobulin, which complexed with pre-existing antibodies in the circulation, and caused removal of antibody as immune complexes were cleared from the circulation over a period of 2 - 3 days.These immune complexes are formed in vivo and relate to thyroid cell destruction, but rarely cause immune complex disease.

T lymphocyte suppressor cell function was studied by a Con-A stimulation assay and by a pre-incubation assay, and was found deficient in patients with active Graves' disease, and patients toxic under treatment, whereas many cured patients had normal suppressor cell function. T- Cells from patients with Graves' disease fail to suppress immunoglobulin synthesis normally in a pokeweed mitogen stimulated system in vitro, and fail to suppress allogeneic B-Cells. Normal T-Cells are able to suppress Graves' B-Cell mediated IgG synthesis, again indicating an abnormality of T lymphocyte suppressor function in active Graves' disease. Recently we have enumerated T lymphocyte subsets using monoclonal antibodies. In patients with active Graves' disease, there is a relative deficiency of suppressor cells identified by the OKT_8 antibody.

Patients with Graves' disease have a genetic propensity to form antibodies and may have hereditary abnormalities in suppressor function. Suppressor cell abnormalities are most obvious during thyrotoxic Graves' disease, but tend to return toward normal when the disease is controlled. Thyrotoxicosis itself may exacerbate autoimmunity.

ACKNOWLEDGEMENTS

Supported by United States Public Health Service Grants AM-13377 and AM-27384

REFERENCES

Adams, D.D., Kennedy T.H., 1967 Occurrence of thyrotoxicosis of gamma globulin which protects LATS from neutralization by an extract of thyroid gland. J Clin Endocrinol Metab 27:173

Aoki, N., De Groot, L.J., 1979 Lumphocyte blastogenic response to human thyroglobulin in Graves' disease, Hashimoto's thyroiditis, and metastatic thyroid cancer.

Clin Exp Immunol 38:523
Antel, J.P., Arnason, B.G.W., Medof, M.E., 1978 Suppressor cell function in multiple sclerosis. Correlation with clinical disease activity. Ann Neurol 5:338
Aoki, N., Pinnamaneni, K.M., De Groot, L.J., 1979 Studies on suppressor cell function in thyroid diseases. J Clin Endocrinol Metab 48:803
Beck, K., Lumholtz, B., Nerup, J., Thomsen, M., Platz, P., Ryder, L.P., Svejgaard, A., Sierbaek-nielsen, K., Hansen, J.M., Larson, J.H.,1977 HLA antigen in Graves' disease. Acta Endocrinol (Copenhagen) 86:150
Bresnhian, B., Jasin, H.E., 1977 Suppressor function of peripheral blood monocuclear cells in normal individuals and in patients with systemic lupus erythematosus. J Clin Invest 59:106
Burnet, F.M., 1959 The Clonal theory of acquired immunity. Cambridge University Press, Cambridge
Clague, R., Mukhtar,E.D., Pyle, G.A., Nutt, J, Clark, F., Scott, M., Evered, D., Rees Smith, B., Hall, R., 1976 Thyroid-stimulating immunoglobulins and the control of thyroid function. J Clin Endocrinol Metab 43:550
Chopra J., Solomon, D.H., Chopra, U., Yoshihara, E., Teresaki P.I., Smith, F., 1977 Abnormalities in thyroid function in relatives of patients with Graves' disease and Hasimoto's thyroiditis. Lack of correlation with inheritance of HLA-B_8.J Clin Endocrinol Metab 45:45
Chattopadhyay,C., Chattopadhyay, H., Natvig, J.B., Mellbye, O.J., 1979 Rheumatoid synovial lymphocytes lack Concavalin A activated suppressor cell activity. Scand J Immunol 10:479
Doniach, D., Roitt, I.M., 1957 Autoimmunity in Hashimoto's disease and its implications. J Clin Endocrinol Metab 17:1293
Doniach, D., 1975 Humoral and genetic aspects of thyroid autoimmunity. Clin Endocrinol Metab 4:267
Doniach, D., Bottazzo, G.F., Russell, R.C.G., 1979 Goitrous autoimmune thyroiditis (Hashimoto's disease) Clin Endocrinol Metab 8:63
Doniach, D., Nilsson, L.R., Roitt I.M., 1965 Autoimmune thyroiditis in children and adolescents. II. Immunological correlations and parent study. Acta Ped Scand 54:260
DeGroot, L.J.,Carey,C., Skosey, C., Pinnamaneni, K.M., Mariotti, S., Barsano, C.P., 1980 The development of clinical thyrotoxicosis: Pre-Graves' disease. In: Pinchera A (ed) Autoimmune aspects of endocrine disorders. Academic Press, New York.

Fenzi, G., Hashizume,K., Roudebush, C.P., DeGroot, L.J., 1979 Changes in thyroid stimulating immunoglobulins during antithyroid therapy. J Clin Endocrinol Metab 48:572
Friedman, I.M.,Fialkow, P.J., 1978 The genetics of Graves' disease. Clin Endocrinol Metab 7:47
Farid, N.R., Von Westarp, C., Row, V.V., Volpé, R., 1974 Studies of cell-mediated immunity (CMI) in relatives of patients with Graves' disease. J Clin Endocrinol Metab 39:779
Ford, D., Knight, J.G., Reeve, J.K., Stewart, R.D.H., 1976 Histocompatibility antigens in Graves' disease. Aust N Z J Med 6:297
Farid, N.R., Sampson, L., Noel, E.P., Barnard, J.M., Mandeville, R.,Larsen, B., Marshall, W.H., 1979 A study of human leukocyte D locus related antigens in Graves' disease J Clin Invest 63:108
Farid, N.R., Sampson, L., Moens, H., Barnard, J.M., 1981 The association of goitrous autoimmune thyroiditis with HLA-Dr5. Tissue Antigens 17:265
Grumet, F.C., Payne, R.O., Konishi, J., Kriss, J.P., 1974 HLA antigens as markers for disease susceptibility and autoimmunity in Graves' disease. J Clin Endocrinol Metab 39:1115
Gonzalez,R.L., Dan, P.C., Splitler, L.E., 1979 Altered regulation of mitogen responsiveness by suppressor cells in multiple sclerosis. Clin Exp Immunol 36:78
Horvath, F., Teague, P., Gaffney, E.F., Mars, D.R., Fuller, T.J., 1979 Thyroid antigen associated immune complex glomerulonephritis in Graves' disease. Am J Med 67:901
Jordan, S.C., Johnston, W.H., Bergtein J.M., 1978 Immune complex glomerulonephritis mediated by thyroid antigens. Arch Pathol Lab Med 102:530
Jordan, S.C., Buckingham, B., Sakai, R., Olson, D., 1981 Studies of immune complex glomerulonephritis mediated by human thyroglobulin. N Eng J Med 304:1212
Kalman, K., Erdei, I., Sandor, P., Fazakas, S., Leövey, A., 1978 Leukocyte migration test for the study of immune reactivity in cases of Graves' disease associated with infiltrative ophthalmopathy. Acta Med Acad Sci Hung 35:29
Kalderon, A.E, Bogaars, H.A., 1977 Immune complex deposits in Graves' disease and Hashimoto's thyroiditis. Am J Med 63:729
Konishi, J., Herman, M.M., Kriss, J.P., 1974 Binding of thyroglobulin and thyroglobulin-antithyroglobulin immune complex to extraocular muscle membrane. Endocrinology 95:434

Lamki, L, Row, V.V., Volpé, R., 1973 Cell-mediated immunity in Graves' disease and Hashimoto's thyroiditis as shown by the demonstration of migration inhibition factors (MIF) J Clin Endocrinol Metab 36:358

Mariotti, S.,Pinchera, A., Marcocci, C., Vitti, P., Urbano, C., Chiovata, L., Tosi, M., Baschieri, L., 1979 Solubilization of human thyroid microsomal antigen. J Clin Endocrinol Metab 48:207

Manley, S.W., Bourke, J.R., Hawker, R.W., 1974 The thyrotropin receptor in guinea pig thyroid homogenate: interaction with the long-acting thyroid stimulator. J Endocrinol. 61:437

Mariotti, S., DeGroot, L.J., Scarborough, D., Medof, M.E., 1979 Study of circulating immune complexes in thyroid diseases. Comparison of Raji cell radioimmunoassay and specific thyroglobulin-antithyroglobulin radioassay. J Clin Endocrinlo Metab 49:679

McKenzie, J.M., 1967 The long- acting thyroid stimulator: Its role in Graves' disease. Recent Prog Horm Res 23:1

Mariotti, S., Kaplan, E.L., Medof, M.E., DeGroot, L.J., 1980 Circulating thyroid antigen-antibody immune complex. Thyroid research VIII -- Proceedings of the Eighth International Thyroid Congress, Sydney, Australia, February 3 - 8, 1980

McLachan, S.M., Bird, A.G., Weetman, A.P., Rees Smith, B., Hall, R., 1981 Use of plaque assays to study thyroglobulin autoantibody synthesis by human peripheral blood lymphocytes Scand J Immunol (in press)

O'Donnell, J., Trokoudes, K., Silverberg, J., Row, V., Volpé, R., 1978 Thyrotropin displacement activity of serum immunoglobulins from patients with Graves' disease. J Clin Endocrinol Metab 46:770

Okita, N., Kidd, A., Row, V.V., Volpé, R., 1980 Sensitization of T-lymphocytes in Graves' and Hashimoto's diseases. J Clin Endocrinol Metab 51: 316

Ohtaki, S., Endo, Y., Horinouchi, K., Yoshitake, S., Ishikawa, E, 1981 Circulating thyroglobulin-antithyroglobulin immune complex in thyroid diseases using enzyme-linked immunoassays. J. Clin Endocrinol Metab 52:239

O' Regan, S., Fong, J.S.C., Kaplan, B.S., DeChadarevian, J.P., Lapointe, N,, Drummond, K.N., 1976 Thyroid antigen-antibody nephritis. Clin Immunol Immunopathol 6:341

Ploth, D.W., Fitz, A., Schnetzler, D., Seidenfeld, J., Wilson, C.B., 1978 Thyroglobulin- antithyroglobulin immune complex glomerulonephritis complicating radioiodine therapy Clin Immunol Immunopathol 9:327

Pacini, F., 1981 Studies of T and B cell interaction in patients with Graves' disease. Eleventh Annual Meeting of the European Thyroid Association, September 1981 Pisa, Italy (abstract)

Roitt, I.M., Doniach, D., Campbell, P.N., Hudson, R.V., 1956 Autoantibodies in Hashimoto's disease (lymphadenoid goiter).Lancet 2:820

Rose,N.R., Witebsky, E., 1956 Studies on organ specifity. V. Changes in the thyroid glands of rabbits following active immunization with rabbit thyroid extracts J Immunol 76:417

Roitt, I.M., Doniach, D., 1967 A reassessment of studies on the aggregation of thyroid autoimmunity in families of thyroiditis patients. Clin Exp Immunol 2:727

Smith, B.R., Hall, R., 1974 Thyroid-stimulating immunoglobulins in Graves' disease. Lancet 2:427

Sakane, T, Steinberg, A.D., Green, I., 1978 Studies of immune functions of patients with systemic lupus erythematosus. I. Dysfunction of suppressor T-cell activity related to impaired generation of, rather than response to, suppressor cells. Arthritis Rheumatol 21:657

Sridama, V., Pacini, F., DeGroot, L.J., 1981 Decreased suppressor T lymphocytes in autoimmune thyroid diseases detected by monoclonal antibodies. J Clin Endocrinol Metab (in press)

Tunbridge, W.M.G., Evered, D.C., Hall, R., Appleton, D., Brewis, M., Clark, F., Grimley-Evans, J., Young, E., Bird, J., Smith, P.A., 1977 The spectrum of thyroid disease in a community: The Whickham Survey. Clin Endocrinol (Oxf) 7:481

Tamai, H., Ohsako, N., Takeno, K., Fukino, O., Takahashi, H., Kumagai, L.F., Nagataki, S., 1980 Changes in thyroid function in euthyroid subjects with a family history of Graves'disease: A follow-up study of 69 patients. J Clin Endocrinol Metab 51:5

Takeda, Y., Kriss, J.P., 1977 Radiometric measurement of thyroglobulin-antithyroglobulin immune complex in human serum. J Clin Endocrinol Metab 44:46

Werner, S.C., Wegelius, O., Fierer, J.A., Hsu, K.C., 1972 Immunoglobulin (E, M, G,) and complement in the connective tissues of the thyroid in Graves' disease. N Engl J Med 287:421

Whittingham, S., Morris, P.J., Martin, F.I.R., 1975 HLA-8: A genetic link with thyrotoxicosis. Tissue Antigens 6:23

Weissel, M., Hofer, R., Zasmeta, H., Mays, W.R., 1980 HLA-Dr and Hashimoto's thyroiditis. Tissue Antigens 16:256

Weiss, I., Davies, T.F., 1981 Identification and quantitation of human thyroglobulin antibodies (h Tg-Ab)-secreting immunocytes in autoimmune thyroid disease. Sixty-third Annual Meeting of the Endocrine Society Program and Abstracts (Abstract 1037)

Waldmann, T.A., Blaese, R.M., Broder, S., Krakauer, R.S., 1978 Disorders of suppressor immunoregulatory cells in the pathogenesis of immunodeficiency and autoimmunity. Ann Intern Med 88:226

Weigle, W.O., Nakamura, R.B., 1969 Perpetuation of autoimmune thyroiditis and production of secondary renal lessions following periodic injections of aqueous preparations of altered thyroglobulin. Clin Exp Immunol 4:645

New Concepts in Thyroid Disease, pages 23–44

ROLE OF CIRCULATING THYROID HORMONES AND LOCAL MECHANISMS IN DETERMINIG THE CONCENTRATION OF T_3 IN VARIOUS TISSUES

J.Enrique Silva

Howard Hughes Medical Institute Laboratory and
Brigham and Women´s Hospital,Dept, of Medicine
Harvard Medical School of Boston,Mass.U.S.A.

By definition an endocrine gland is an organ-or a tissue-that secretes its product directly in the circulation to be delivered to the other tissues.The concentration of the product in the circulation has always been considered a reflection of its supply to the cells.While this is still essentially a well accepted and well supported concept, a better knowledge of the physiology and biochemistry of the hormones has evidenced that the situation may be far more complex in many cases.For example,testosterone,the main secretory product of the Leydig cells in the testis is not ultimately responsible for the biological action in the cells of the various target tissues.In most responsive tissues it is transformed into a more active form,dihydrotestosterone. Although the concentration of testosterone in the serum reflects the potential supply of the more active end product to the tissues,it does not necessarily reflect its actual concentration,since the rate of conversion in the cells may vary from tissue to tissue,from one individual to another and even in the same tissue,depending on a number of different variables.Over the last decade,the study of thyroid hormone physiology has also revealed that the relationship between plasma and tissue concentrations is much more complicated than it was originally suspected. In this chapter we will discuss our present understanding on this subject and the implications that these new concepts have in the understanding and management of the patients suffering thyroid disorders.

Ever since the discovery of 3,5,3' l-triiodothyronine (T_3) by Gross and Pitt Rivers in 1952,the evidence that this substance accounts for most-nearly all- the biological potency of the thyroid gland secretion has acumulated and this concept is now widely accepted(Larsen,P.R.,1981).Most of this evidence has been reviewed and summarized in the chapter on Adaptation to Iodine Deficiency in this book.

Although during the 1960's some reports(Tata,J.R.,1966, Tommaselli,A.,1965)suggested that thyroid hormone expression was mediated through changes in protein synthesis by a nuclear action,the concept developed rapidly only after specific high affinity and low capacity receptors were described in the cell nuclei from tissues responsive to thyroid hormone(Oppenheimer,J.H.,1973).Today the nucleus as the site of initiation of thyroid hormone action is also a widely accepted concept,although other possible mechanisms of action cannot be excluded.The evidence supporting thisconcept is summarized in Table 1.The fact that these receptors have at least 10 times higher affinity for T_3 than for thyroxine (T_4)in vitro (Oppenheimer,J.H.,1973, Degroot,L.J.,1974)and that in vivo 10% of less of the nuclear iodothyroninefound the liver and kidney is T_4(Surks,M.I., 1977)is consistent with the idea that at a cellular level ultimately,the hormone is T_3(see also chapter 6).Accordingly we will start by focussing our discussion on the regulation of nuclear T_3 concentration.

After unraveling the existence of nuclear T_3 binding sites that were saturable (Oppenheimer,J.H.,1972-Koerner,J. 1974)Oppenheimer and colleagues studied the kinetics of the exchange with serum(Oppenheimer,J.H.1974).From the time course of nuclear occupancy after a pulse of labelled T_3(T_3*) and the simultaneous changes of serum T_3*levels,they developed a model based on one previously used for the analysis of albumin kinetics in man (Pearson,J.D.,1958).This model is schematically represented in Fig.1A. After a pulse of T_3* ,at tracer concentrations,serum T_3exchanges rapidly with cytoplasm whereas the specific activity of nuclear T_3 rises more slowly.At some point in time,the nuclear specific activity is maximal and transiently the rate of change of nuclear T_3* is 0,that is,the velocity of binding equals that of dissociation.Since by definition a tracer injection of T_3 has not disturbed the system which is assumed to be in steady state,ie,the velocities of dissociation and association of endogenous T_3 from the nucleus are equal,it results that the specific activity of plasma T_3 and nuclear $T_3$are equal ,and therefore the concentration of T_3in the

TABLE 1

Evidence Favoring the Nucleus as The Site of Initiation of Thyroid Hormone

Action

- -- The earliest detectable effect in the liver after the injection of T_3 is the incorporation of ^{14}C-orotic acid into nuclear RNA.
- -- Protein synthesis inhibitors can block a number of physiological effects of thyroid hormone
- -- Increases in specific messanger RNA´s have been detected after the injection of thyroid hormone
- -- There are specific high affinity low capacity binding sites for triiodothyronine in those tissues responsive to thyroid hormone.Non-responsive tissues lack these receptors.
- -- The biological response to thyroid hormone analogs correlate very well with their affinity for these binding sites
- -- A number of responses to thyroid hormone have been correlated chronologically and quantitatively with thyroid hormone binding to these receptors
- -- Although receptors have been found in other subcellular fractions,their binding characteristics, tissue distribution and time course of binding have not been correlated to biological responses to thyroid hormone as the nuclear receptors have.

nucleus can be calculated from the plasma specific activity. This short interval of time(theoretically a time point),is called equilibrium time piont,tm.These studies were done in the liver and subsequently the application of the model was extended to other tissues(Oppenheimer,J.H.,1974).The tm ranged from 20-30 min (kidney-liver) to 3 hours (brain).With measurements done at the appropriate time after the injection of T_3* they calculated the nuclear T_3 content in several tissues at endogenous T_3 levels.By saturation techniques they also estimated the maximal capacity of binding T_3(MBC)of nuclei from all tissues (Oppenheimer,J.H.,1974).The results indicated that the nuclears receptors were about 50% occupied at physiological concentrations of T_3. Since the implication was that the affinity of the receptors did not differ from one tissue to another, it resulted that in any tissue the nuclear T_3 content was well reflected by the plasma concentration of the hormone.

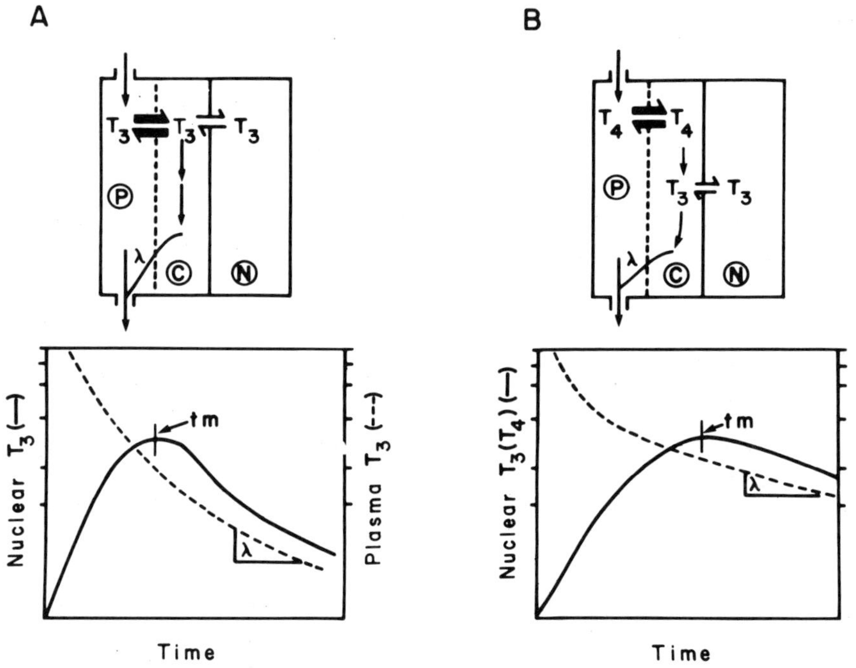

Fig 1.-A. Schematic representation of plasma-cytoplasma-nuclear exchange of T_3 after the intravenous injection of bolus of labelled hormone.

B. Schematic representation of plasma-cytoplasma exchange of T_4 and nuclear binding of T_3 produced from T_4 in the cell, after an intravenous bolus of labelled T_4.

This model of thyroid hormone action fitted very well most experimental and clinical observations, namely, that the thyroid status correlated nicely with serum T_3 levels.The best examples,discussed in Chapter 6,were iodine deficiency and other situations of decreased thyroid reserve,like early stages of Hashimoto's thyroiditis,and Graves' disease patients treated with radioactive iodine who have low serum T_4 or PBI and yet they are euthyroid.The euthyroidism could well be accounted for by the normal level of T_3 in excellent agreement with the model discussed.However a number of discrepancies were apparent.The same iodine deficient animals metabolically euthyroid (Silva,J.E.,1972)and,accordingly with normal T_3have elevated TSH (Fukuda,H.,1975).Similar observations were made in iodine deficient humansliving in endemic goiter areas (Chopra,L.J.,1975 -Goslings,B.,1972) and in individuals with early stages of hypothyroidism (Larsen,P.R.,1981).Patients with hepatic cirrhosis(Chopra I.J.,1974)or other non-thyroidal illnesses(Bermudez,F.,1975) on the other hand,have normal T_4,low T_3 and normal TSH.Larsen and Frumess(Larsen,P.R.,1977)studied several effects of thyroid hormone in thyroidectomized rats treated with either T_4 or T_3.They used propylthiouracil (PTU) to block the conversion of T_4 to T_3.This drug almost completely blunted the effect of T_4 on the liver enzyme alfa-glycerophasphate dehydrogenase (alfa-GPD) but body weigh gained (growth) and the suppression of TSH in response to T_4 were minimally affected by PTU.Obviously the pituitary seemed to be responsive to T_4 serum levels.

There were many possible ways to explain these observations.One of them was that the pituitary had specific and unique receptors for T_4,either in the cell nuclei or elsewhere in the cell.Other was that T_4 was converted to T_3 in the pituitary,but this mechanism seemed unlikely based on the failure of PTU to block the suppresive effect of T_4 on TSH secretion (Larsen,P.R.,1977) and the failure of some early attempts to demonstrate in vitro T_4 to T_3 conversion in pituitary homogenates (Galton,V.A. 1976).Our early studies showed that the suppression by T_3 was very closely related both chronologically and quantitatively to nuclear T_3 content after a single dose of 70 ng/100 g of T_3 was given to thyroidectomized rats (Silva,J.E.,1977)(see also Chapter 6), so that,at least the T_3 induced TSH suppression seemed mediated by nuclear receptors.When T_4 was given to these animals,TSH suppression could be entirely accounted for by the amount of T_3 generated and present in the nucleus of anterior pituitary cells (Silva,J.E.,1977).No significant amounts of T_4 could be detected in the nucleus of these cells

(Silva,J.E.,1978).Since there was no elevation of serum T_3 after T_4 injection in these acute experiments and since this dose of T_4 did not facilitate the entrance of T_3 into the cell nuclei from the plasma,we concluded that the T_3 found after T_4 had been produced in the pituitary (Silva,J. E.,1977).It thus seems that intrapituitary T_3,at least in these experimental conditions,could not be predicted from the serum level of T_3.This was subsequently demonstrated in experiments where two small non-saturating doses of $^{131}I-T_3$ were injected along with a small dose of $^{125}I-T_4$ to thyroidectomized rats (Silva,J.E.,1978).While at a given level of serum T_3 the same fraction of kidney,liver and pituitary T_3 nuclear receptors were occupied,the T_4 added significant greater amounts of T_3 to the pituitary nuclei than to liver and kidney nuclei(Silva,J.E.,1978).The amount of T_3 derived from serum T_3 was comparable in all 3 tissues but the total intracellular T_3 was not predictable from the serum T_3 level since the T_4 made a significantly greater contribution to the intrapituitary nuclear T_3 than to that of the liver and kidney.Obviously,one could not predict the endogenous T_3 levels in all tissues based on the serum T_3 specific activity and the nuclear concentration of T_3* because this approach did not take into consideration the hormone produced in the tissue from T_4.Neither could one do it from serum T_4 and T_3,since the fraction of nuclear T_3 derived from tissue T_4 was different from one tissue to another.

In order to estimate which was the contribution of each source in various tissues in the euthyroid rat,we used an approach similar to that previously used by Oppenheimer et al (Oppenheimer,J.H.,1974)to estimate nuclear T_3 from serum T_4.This is diagramatically illustrated in Fig 1.B. Plasma T_4 equilibrates rapidly with the pituitary (Schadlow,A.R.,1972) and liver and kidney (Oppenheimer,J.H.,1970)and is subsequently metabolized.A fraction of the resulting T_3 would bind to the nuclear receptors and another fraction would probably exit the cell.If a pulse of labelled T_4 is injected to a euthyroid rat,the specific activity of nuclear T_3 is expected to increase slowly.A point in time when the specific activity is maximal and when transiently there is no change in specific activity is expected.Similarly to the model described for plasma-nuclear T_3 exchange,and provided the equilibrium of the system is not disturbed,the velocity of dissociation of endogenous nuclear T_3 derived from this source would be equal to the velocity of association of T_3 derived from T_4 deiodination to the nucleus and,consequently the nuclear content of T_3 derived from this source could be calculated from the specific activity of plasma T_4.We injected $^{125}I-T_4$ and at different times we measured the serum $^{125}I-T_4$ and $^{125}I-T_3$ and nuclear $^{125}I-T_3$ concentrations. Injections of $^{131}I-T_3$ were done with the appropriate timing, and from the concentrations of $^{131}I-T_3$ in the nuclei and in the serum,we calculated the fraction of the total observed nuclear $^{125}I-T_3$ formed elsewhere from the $^{125}I-T_4$ and borne to the tissue under study via plasma.All the nuclear $^{125}I-T_3$ in excess after this correction had to be formed in the tissue.Fig 2 shows a typical experiment done with a rat pituitary.The injection of $^{131}I-T_3$ also allowed us to calculate simultaneously the contribution of endogenous plasma T_3 to nuclear T_3 (Silva,J.E.,1978).The results showed that ,as predicted by Oppenheimer's group (Oppenheimer,J.H., 1974),plasma T_3 accounted for by 40% -50% nuclear occupancy in pituitary,liver and kidney (Silva,J.E.,1978).However, whereas in liver and kidney the nuclear T_3 produced locally from T_4 accounted for only 25 and 10% of nuclear saturation respectively,in the pituitary this source provided T_3 to saturate 40% of the receptors,giving an overall saturation of 80%.As explained and illustrated in Chapter 6,these findings provided a reasonable explanation for those clinical and experimental observations otherwise not explained by the model developed by Oppenheimer and colleagues (Oppenheimer, J.H.,1974-Pearson,J.D.,1958).

With similar methodology we have studied other tissues. In the cerebral cortex , 80% of nuclear T_3 is derived from local T_4 deiodination while in the cerebellum this source provides aproximately 60% of nuclear T_3. Figure 3 shows the time course of nuclear T_3 after injecting $^{131}I-T_3$ and $^{125}I-T_4$ in cerebral contex and cerebellum.The source of nuclear T_3 in all these tissues is summarized in Table 2.

Fig.4 illustrates our current understanding of the sources of intracellular T_3 and the reason why studies based on the injection of T_3 necessarily underestimate the intracellular content of T_3.In all tissues studied so far a fraction of T_3 comes from plasma and another fraction is produced in the tissue from T_4.This fraction does not equilibrate rapidly with plasma T_3 and "stays" in the cell. Thus the injected tracer T_3 entering the cell,will be diluted by the T_3 formed in the cell.Therefore the specific activity of intracellular T_3 always will be less than plasma specific activity and hence quantitations based on the latter will

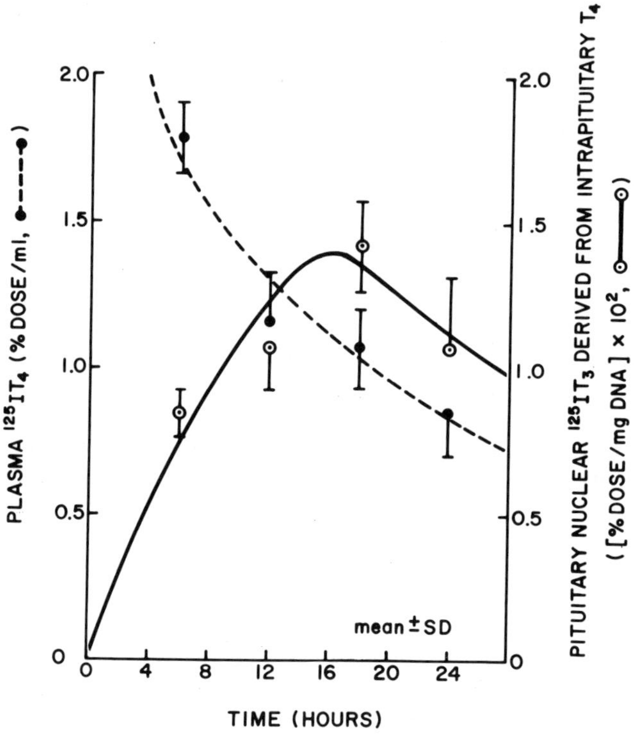

Fig.2.-Time courses of nuclear binding of locally produced ^{125}I-T_3 from ^{125}I-T_4 in the anterior pituitary of euthyroid rats after a bolus injection of ^{125}I-T_4. (From Silva, Dick and Larsen 1978 Endocrinology 103:1196, with permission from the Editor)

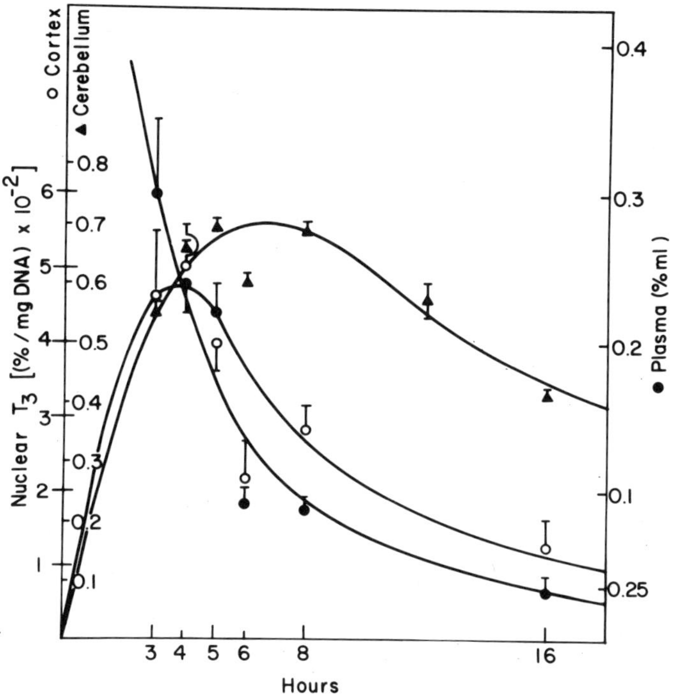

Fig.3. A- Time courses of nuclear binding of $^{125}I-T_3$ in cerebral contaxt and cerebellum after a bolus injection of the tracer to euthyroid rats.

necessarily underestimate intracellular T_3.Likewise,if we wanted to calculate the intracellular T_3 from the specific activity of plasma $^{125}I-T_4$,we would also underestimate it since the T_3* from T_4* in the tissue would be diluted by the unlabelled T_3 entering from plasma.If one injects tracer T_3

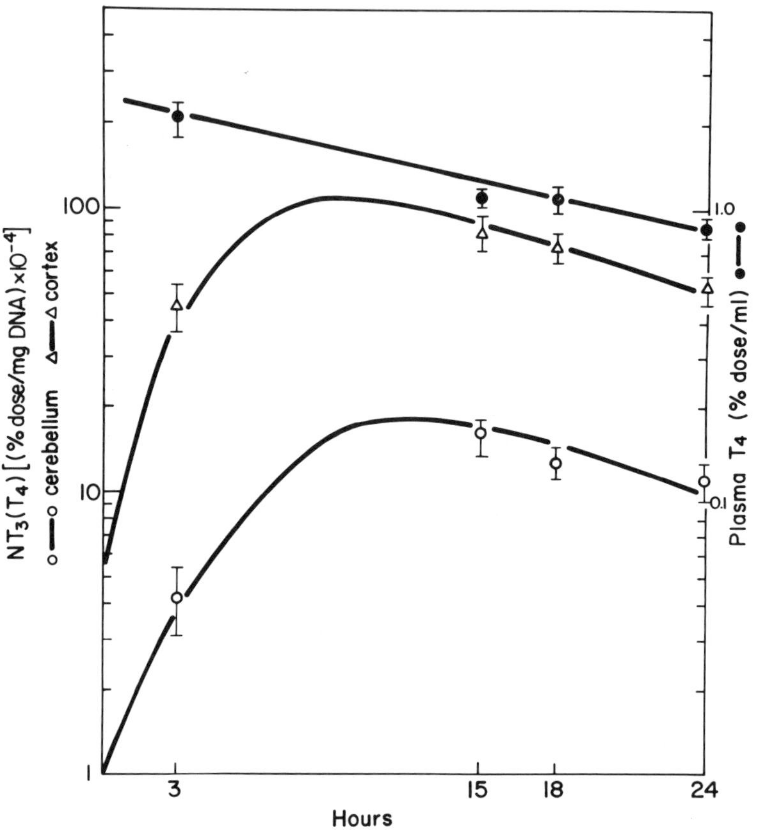

Fig.3. B-Time courses of nuclear binding of locally produced $^{125}I-T_3$ from $^{125}I-T_4$ in cerebral cortex and cerebellum of euthyroid rats after the intravenous injection of a bolus of $^{125}I-T_4$ (From Crantz,Silva and Larsen 1982 Endocrinilogy in press;with permission from the Editor).

and T_4 labelled with different isotopes -as we have-one can estimate the total amount of T_3 in a cell compartment,ie,

Table 2

Relative Contribution of Plasma T_3 ($T_3(T_3)$) and Locally Produced T_3 ($T_3(T_4)$) to Nuclear T_3 in Various Tissues of the Rat

Tissue	$T_3(T_3)$ %	$T_3(T_4)$ %	Overall Saturation %
Liver	75	25	50
Kidney	85	15	50
Pituitary	50	50	80
Cerebellum	50	50	60
Cerebral Cortex	20	80	90

Data from Silva, Dick and Larsen 1978 Endocrinology 103:1196 and Crantz, Silva and Larsen 1982 Endocrinology 110: (In press).

the nucleus, from the specific activity of serum T_3 and serum T_4. The estimation with each tracer is an underestimation, the magnitude of each depending on the magnitude of the other source. For example, in the cerebral cortex where 80% of the T_3 is originated locally (Table 2), studies based on serum T_3 specific activity and tissue T_3* content will tremendously underestimate the intracellular content of T_3 while those based on serum T_4* will minimally do it.

At equilibrium of tracer T_3

$$\frac{N\ T_3^*}{P\ T_3^*} \times P\ T_3(RIA) = N\ T_3(T_3) \qquad 1)$$

$$N\ T_3(T_3) = \text{Total } N\ T_3 - N\ T_3(T_4) \qquad 2)$$

where N T_3 and P T_3 denote nuclear and plasma T_3 respectively; T_3^* is labelled T_3; N T_3^* (T_3), N T_3 (T_3) stand for -respectively- labelled or unlabelled nuclear T_3 derived from plasma;

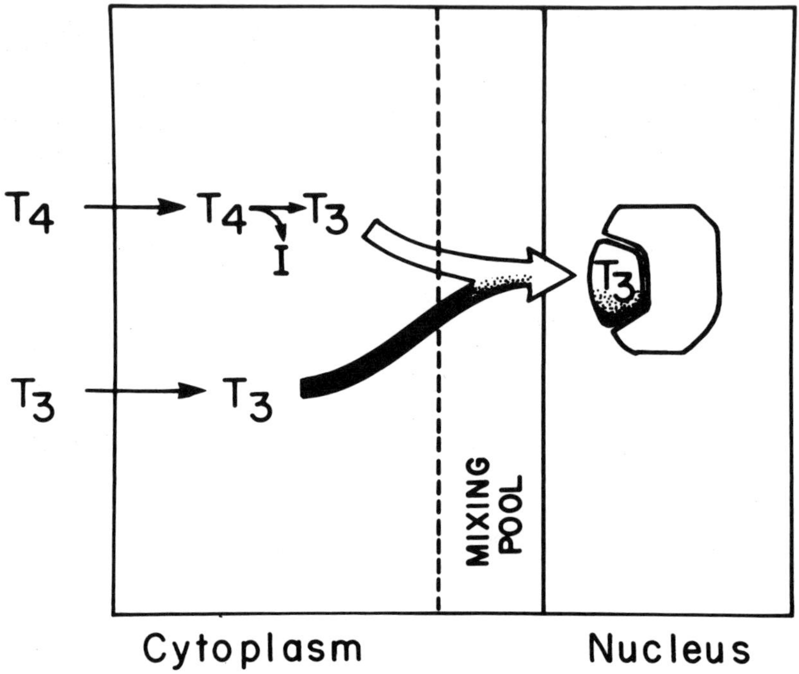

Fig.4.-T_3 binding to nuclear receptors in the cells derives from 2 sources:a) it is transported directly from the plasma and b) is generated in the cell from T_4.If either source is labelled the maximal specific activity of T_3 binding to the nucleus is less than that of the precursor in the plasma because it is deluted by the endogenous unlabelled T_3 from the other source.If labelled T_3 and labelled T_4 with different isotopes are injected with the appropriate timing so as to get the maximal specific activity of each isotope in the nucleus,the relative concentration of isotopes is a reflection of the relative contribution of each source to nuclear T_3.(From Crantz,Silva and Larsen 1982 Endocrinology In press;with permission from the Editor).

$N\ T_3(T_4)$ denotes the nuclear T_3 produced in the tissue from T_4 and $P\ T_3$ RIA is the serum concentration of T_3 measured by radioimmunoassay.These equations simply show that the calculations based on serum T_3 do not take into account the T_3 derived from T_4 in the tissue.

Similarly,at equilibrium of tracer T_4:

$$\frac{N\ T_3^*(T_4^*)}{P\ T_4^*} \times P\ T_4(\text{RIA}) = N\ T_3(T_4) \quad 3)$$

$$N\ T_3(T_4) = \text{Total}\ N\ T_3 - N\ T_3(T_3) \quad 4)$$

where $N\ T_3^*\ (T_4)$ is the labelled T_3 produced from labelled T_4 in situ and all the other symbols are as they have been defined for equations 1 and 2.

By adding equations(1) and (3) and equations (2) and(4) it results that

$$\frac{N\ T_3^*\ (T_3^*)}{P\ T_3^*} \times P\ T_3\ (\text{RIA}) + \frac{N\ T_3^*(T_4^*)}{P\ T_4^*} \times P\ T_4\ (\text{RIA}) = \text{total nuclear } T_3$$

Thus by adding both underestimations we can get the total mass of T_4 in the nucleus and we can calculate which fraction is supplied by each source.This approach has been confirmed by direct measurement of nuclear T_3 by RIA in the pituitary (Silva,J.E.,1978)and in cerebral cortex and cerebellum (in preparation).

As summarizaed in Table 2,these studies have shown that there are tissues like the brain and the pituitary where the intracellular generation T_3 from T_4 is a very or the most important source of T_3,and others like liver, kidney and probably skeletal muscle,myocardium,where the main source of T_3 is plasma T_3.In the latter tissues a fall in serum T_4 is not expected to give rise to a significant depletion of T_3(provided the thyroidal secretion keeps normal the serum T_3 level),but in the pituitary and in the nervous tissue a reduction in serum T_4 is expected to result in a significant fall in tissue T_3.So far,we know that in those low T_4-normal T_3 conditions,mentioned above there is no metabolic evidence of lack of thyroid hormone, but TSH is elevated (Silva,J.E.,1972-Goslings,B.,1972).

Our group has shown that both the pituitary (Larsen,P.R. 1980-Kaplan,M.M.,1980)and the nervous tissue(Kaplan M.M.,1980) can convert enzimatically T_4 to T_3 in vitro confirming in vivo evidence of our own(Silva,J.E.1977-Silva,J.E.1978)and others (Ford,D.H.,1958-Volpert,E.M.,1962).A most interesting finding is that in these tissues the 5'-deiodination of T_4 is elevated in hypothyroidism(Kaplan,M.M.,1980-Kaplan,M.M. 1980) while in the liver this enzyme activity is depressed. The changes in the cerebral cortext are very rapid and marked(Leonard,J.L.,1981),contrasting with other responses of this tissue to thyroid hormone (Silva,J.E.,manuscript in preparation).The divergent response to hypothyroidism of the liver,on the other hand,and the cerebral cortex and pituitary enzyme on the other,suggest that there may be two different enzymes.In agreement with this hypothesis,pretreatment with Propylthiouracil (PTU)does not block T_3 generation from T_4 in the cortex,cerebellum and pituitary while it does decrease the concentration of serum T_3 and the generation of T_3 from T_4 in the liver (Silva,J.E.,in press)in agreement with previous findings (Larsen,P.R.,1977-Oppenheimer,J.H., 1972).Other recent studies carried out in our laboratory (Visser,T.J.,1981)using 125 I-labelled reverse T_3 in the 5' position as substrate for the 5' deiodinase activity,have shown that there are two discernible pathways of 5' deiodination.One has a low Km (2nM)and is sensitive to inhibition by namolar concentrations of T_4(Ki 2 nM) and is not inhibited by PTU;the other has a higher Km (30nM)for reverse T_3 is sensitive to PTU and insensitive to T_4 up to uM concentrations.To date,we have not been able to demonstrate the existence of the low Km-PTU insensitive pathway in the liver and the kidney.The increase induced by hypothyroidism in 5'-deiodinase activity in the cerebral cortex affects solely or more importantly to the low Km-PTU insensitive enzyme(Silva,J.E.,manuscript in preparation-Visser,T.J.,1981)and this effect of hypothyroidism is much more pronounced in the neonatal rat (Kaplan,M.M.,1980-Silva, J.E.,manuscript in preparation)than in the adult rat(Silva, J.E.,manuscript in preparation-Leonard,J.L.,1981).Not only is T_3 formation increased in hypothyroidism but also T_3 degradation is decreased(Silva,J.E.,manuscript in preparation-Leonard,J.L.,1981).Altogether these findings along with the well known need of thyroid hormone of the developing brain and the fact that 60%(cerebellum) to 80%(cerebral cortex)of the T_3 is produced locally from T_4,suggests that the enzyme, the low Km-PTU insensitive one,is a very important locus of regulation of thyroid hormone supply to these tissues. These findings further support the concept that the level of serum T_3 does not necessarily reflect the content of the hormone in the tissues.Both together,serum T_4 and serum T_3 are a better reflection,but the existence of these homeostatic changes at cellular level reveal that the situation is even more complicated.

The discussion that follows shows that the number of factors becoming apparent and that ultimately may have a bearing on T_3 content at the initiation sites in the cell, seems to be increasing.They may have unsuspected effect in some physiological or pathological conditions,although,to date,this is largely speculative.These aditional factors are related to the transport of the thyroid hormone into the cells through membrane-bound mechanisms and to the kinetics of the exchange of thyroid hormones between plasma binding proteins and tissue.

Several groups have shown that there may be an energy dependent saturable transport mechanism of T_3 and T_4 through the membrane of different cells(Pliam,N.B.,1977-Rao,G.S.,1981) These mechanisms are currently under active study and at present it is rather difficult to ascribe a role in physiology or disease.For example,in most of the studies the V max of these transport processes is huge compared to the needs of the cells and the Km(or Kt),thatis the concentration resulting in half of the maximal velocity of transport has been found to be either low (Rao,G.S.,1981) or high(Krenning,E.P.,1978), so that it is difficult to know at what level of the capacity the transport channel works in the animal.There seems to be little or no questions that these mechanisms exist and that they are energy dependent;the major question is which role do they play in health and disease.One group postulates that the level of ATP (Krenning,E.,1980)may regulate the transport of T_4 into the cells and that in conditions like fasting and nonthyroidal illnesses,the low level of cell ATP would determine a reduction in the transport of T_4(T_3 is not that critically dependent on ATP).Although an attractive hypothesis evidence to support it is presently lacking.Another unresolved problem in relation to transmembrance transport,is that diffusion has been shown to occur concomitantly to the active transport,and its relative contribution to the local influx of hormone into the cells in different conditions is not known. Finally, animal studies show that in otherwise physiological conditions, the transport of T_4 or T_3 into the tissues does not saturate even with doses several hundred fold higher than the daily production rate (Schadlow, A.R., 1972-Crantz, F.R., 1982). It is reasonable to conclude that under physiological conditions membrane transport is not a rate limiting step in the availability of thyroid hormone to the cell. Since transportation of T_4 has been shown to be energy dependent (Krenning, E., 1980) and it can also be interfered by some humoral factors evidenced in non-thyroidal illnesses (Chopra, I.J., 1979-Oppenheimer, J.H., 1981), it is possible that in conditions like fasting and a variety of non-thyroidal illnesses, the fractional transport rate into the cell is decreased. Even so, considering other concomitant changes such as a decrease in plasma binding, reduction in the rate of metabolism in the tissue, i e, T_4 to T_3 conversion, the concentration of T_4 in the cell may not be substantially altered despite the reduction in the fractional transport rate as determined in vitro.

Dr. Pardrige's studies (Pardrige, W.M., 1981) on plasma-tissue exchange have challenged the long standing concept on the relevance of the in vitro measured thyroid hormone concentration. He has developed a more dynamic view in which other factors are taken into consideration. These factors are the rate of dissociation of T_4 and T_3 from plasma binding proteins, the time of exposure of the cells of a given tissue to the hormone, as reflected by the capillary transit time, and the diffusibility of the hormone through the membrane into the cell. Thus, the liver capillary transit time is approximately 5 seconds while that of the brain is only 1 second. The half time of dissociation of T_3 from albumin is $<$ 1 second and from TBPA (the rat has no TBG) is about 4 seconds. The corresponding figures for T_4 are 1 sec and 8 sec respectively. Therefore, in the rat T_3 is widely available for liver while only that bound to albumin is available for the brain. Basically only the albumin-bound T_4 is available for both tissues (Pardrige, W.M., 1981). This explains why the fractional transfer of T_3 from plasma to liver is much greater than that from plasma to brain and also greater than the fractional rates of T_4 to both tissues. Another important implication of these studies is that the fraction of hormone available to the tissues is greater than the free fraction as determined by equilibrium dialysis. Consistent with this view they have recently communicated that T_4 diluted in serum from sick patients,where the dialysable fraction as determined in vitro is higher than in healthy controls,is not more available to the tissues than that diluted in normal human serum(Pardrige,W.M.1981).Altogether these studies emphasize the role of circulatory factors,potentially subject to local regulatory mechanisms,in the availability of thyroid hormone to the cells.

In brief,we have reviewed recent evidence showing the complexity of the relationship of the intracellular thyroid hormone T_3 with its plasma precursor T_4 and with the pre-formed plasma hormone.The level of serum T_3 does not reflect necessarily the intracellular concentrations of the hormones in all tissues.It does it fairly well for tissues like liver, kidney,heart,skeletal muscle whose major source of T_3 is the plasma,but it does not in those like pituitary and brain that depend heavily on the intracellular generation of T_3 from T_4.Here,T_3 concentration is betterr reflected by both serum T_4 and T_3.But since the capacity of these tissues to generate T_3 from T_4 increases in hypothyroidism one cannot assume that the concentration of T_3 from T_4 will bear a simple linear relationship with serum T_4.The situation is more complex since local factors derived from physiological responses or disease,could interfere with the availability of T_4 and/or T_3 to the tissues-through transport mechanisms and circulatory conditions for tissue-plasma exchange-or with the homeostatic changes in 5'-deiodination of T_4 or 5-deiodination of T_3.

This review has intended to be a güide to answer a number of questions raised about patient management.Typical questions are:What to use for hormone replacement in hypothyroidism T_4,T_3 or combinations thereof? How can TSH secretion be better and safely suppressed in patients with thyroid carcinoma? What is the meaning of a low serum T_4 in newborns of moderate iodine deficient areas? How could a patient treated for Graves' disease with antithyroid drugs have an elevated serum T_3 and yet low T_4,high TSH and be clinically slightly hyperthyroid? Our answer to these questions should flow out of this analyses,although we are aware of the complexity of the situation and the possibility of as yet unknown factors that might change our present interpretations.Thus,we think that the replacement therapy for hypothyroid patients should be T_4.With this substance normal plasma levels of both T_4 and T_3 are obtainable and the supply of T_3 will be normal in all tissues,those more heavily dependent on T_4 for T_3 generation and those mostly dependent on serum T_3 concentration.The amount of T_3 generated will be subjected to all those homeostatic mechanisms described above,as normally is,which would not happen with fixed combinations of T_4 and T_3.Similarly T_4 seems more appropriate to suppress TSH secretion in patients with thyroid carcinoma because it can provide maximal amounts of T_3 for the anterior pituitary without elevating substantially the plasma concentration of T_3.To supress TSH with T_3 necessarily requires to elevate the serum T_3 concentration,at least, transiently,to hyperthyroid levels.The low level of T_4 seen in cord blood of newborns from iodine deficient areas indicate that the brain T_3 content might have been significantly decreased (certainly the pituitary has,since TSH is elevated in these newborns)at some point during development,although studies showing an increase in 5' deiodination of T_4 suggest that there may be a compensation. A patient with Graves' disease on antithyroid drugs may have a significant depletion to thyroidal iodine to produce mostly T_3.If the blockade is not complete,the serum concentration may be significantly albeit not markedly elevated,but serum T_4 may be reduced bellow normal limits. The total amount of T_3 derived from the combined levels of serum T_3 and T_4 in the pituitary may not be enough to saturate the nuclei of the thyrotrophs to normal levels,but the elevated concentration of T_3 in the plasma will result in hyperthyroid levels of saturation in liver,kidney,heart, muscle nuclei and these are the tissues giving rise to most of the symptoms of hyperthyroidism.The growth of the goiter derived from the elevated TSH may erroneously lead the physician to think that the patient needs more antithyroid drugs.

ACKNOWLEDGEMENTS

The work presented here has been supported mostly by the grant AM 18616 from the National Institute of Health.I am deeply indebted to Dr.P.Reed Larsen,principal investigator of this grant,under whose direction the work that constitutes the core of this presentation has been done.I also would like to acknowledge the careful technical assistance of T.E. Dick S.Mellen and G.Weiss,the secretarial work of Faith Baldwin,and the collaboration of Drs. M.M. Kaplan,and J.L. Leonard.

REFERENCES

Bardin,C.W.,Paulsen,A.C.(1981) The testes.In Textbook of Endocrinology R.H.Williams Editor Saunders Philadelphia, page 293.

Bermudez,F., Surks,M.I.,and Oppenheimer,J.H. 1975 High incidence of decreased serum triiodothyronine concentration with nonthyroidal disease.J.Clin.Endocrinol.Metab 41:27

Crantz,F.R.,Silva,J.E.,and Larsen P.R. 1982 Analysis of the sources and quantity of 3,5,3'-triiodothyronine specifically bound to nuclear receptors in rat cerebral cortex and cerebellum.Endocrinology In press

Chopra,L.J.,Hersham,J.M.,and R.W.Hornabrook.1975 Thyroid hormone and thyrotropin levels in subjects from endemic goiter regions of New Guinea.J.Clin.Endocrinol Metab.40:326

Chopra,I.J.,Solomon,D.H.,Chopra,V.,Young,R.T.,Chua-Teco,G.N. 1974 Alterations in circulating thyroid hormones and thyrotropic in hepatic cirrhosis:Evidence for euthyroidism despite subnormal serum triiodothyronine.J.Clin Endocrinol Metab 39:501

Chopra,I.J.,Chau-Teco,G.N.,Nguyen,A.H.and Solomon D.H. 1979 In search of an inhibitor of thyroid hormone binding to serum porteins in nonthyroidal illnesses.J.Clin.Endocrinol. Metab 49:63

Degroot,L.J. and Strausser,J.L. 1974 Binding of T_3 in rat liver nuclei.Endocrinology 95:74

Ford,D.H.,and Gross,J. 1958 The metabolism of 131 I-labelled thyroid hormones in the hypophysis and brain of the rabbit, Endocrinology 62:416

Fukuda,H.,Yasuda,N.,Greer,M.A.,and Greer,S.E. 1975 Changes in Plasma Thyroxine,triiodothyronine and TSH during adaptation to iodine deficiency in the rat Endocrinology 97:307

Galton,V.A. 1976 The metabolism of thyroid hormones in rat pituitary.In:Thyroid Research (eds) Robbins,J.,and Braverman,L.E. Proceedings of the seventh international thyroid conference.Excerpta Medica,Amsterdam,pp 251-254

Ghabbi,J.,and Torresani,J. 1979 High affinity thyroxine binding to purified rat liver plasma membranes.Biochem. Biophys.Res. Comm.88:170

Goslings,B.,Djokomoeljanto,R.?Docter,van Hardeveld van,C., Hennemann,G.,Smeenk,D.,and Querido,A.1972 Hypothyroidism in an area of endemic goiter and cretinism in Central Java, Indonesia J.Clin.Endocrinol Metab 44:481

Gross,J.,Pitt-Rivers,R.(1952)The identification of 3,5,3' I-triiodothyronine in human plasma.Lancet 1:439

Kaplan,M.M. 1980 Thyroxine 5'-monodeiodination in rat anterior pituitary homogenates.Endocrinology 106:567
Kaplan,M.M. and Yaskoski,K.A. 1980.Phenolic and tyrosyl ring iodothyronine deiodination in rat brain homogenates.J. Clin.Invest.66:551
Krenning,E.P.,Docter,R.,Bernard,H.F.,Visser,T.J. and Hennemann,G.1978 Active transport of triiodothyronine(T_3) into isolated rat liver cells.FEBS Letters 91:113
Krenning,E.,Docter,R.,Bernard,B.,Visser,T.J.and Hennemann,G. 1980 Regulation of the active transport of 3,3',5-triiodothyronine into primary cultured rat hepatocytes by ATP.FEBS Letters 119:279
Koerner,J.,M.L.surks and J.H.Oppenheimer.1974 In vitro demonstration of specific triiodothyronine bindings sites in rat liver nuclei.J.Clin.Endocrinol Metab.38:706
Larsen,P.R.,Silva,J.E.and Kaplan,M.M. 1981 Relationships between circulating and intracellular thyroid hormones: Physiological and clinical implications.Endo.Rev 2:87-102
Larsen,P.R.,and Frumess,R.D. 1977 Comparison of the biological effects of thyroxine and triiodothyronine in the rat 100:980-988
Larsen,P.R.,Bavli,S.Z.,Castonguay,M.and Jove R.1980 Direct radioimmunoassay of nuclear 3,5,3'-triiodothyronine in rat anterior pituitary J.Clin Invest 65:675
Leonard,J.L.,Kaplan,M.M.,Visser,T.J.,Silva,J.E.and Larsen P.R. 1981 Cerebral cortex responds rapidly to thyroid hormones Science 214:571
Oppenheimer,J.H.,D.Koerner,H.L.Scwartz and M.I.Surks 1972 Specific nuclear triiodothyronine binding sites in rat liver and kidney J.Clin.Endocrinol Metab 35:330
Oppenheimer,J.H.,H.L.Scwartz,W.Dillman and M.I.Surks 1973 Effects of thyroid hormone analogues on the displacement of 125 I-L-triiodothyronine from hepatic and heart nuclei in vivo:Possible relationship to hormonal activity.Biochem Biophys.Res.Comm.55;N.3,544
Oppenheimer,J.H.,H.L.Schwartz,Koerner,D.and M.I.Surks. 1974 Limited binding capacity sites for L-triiodothyronine in rat liver nuclei:nuclear-cytoplasmic interrelation, binding constants,and cross-reactivity with L-thyroxine J.Cli Invest 53:768
Oppenheimer,J.H.,Schwartz,H.L.and Surks,M.I. 1974 Tissue differences in the concentration of triiodothyronine nuclear binding sites in the rat:liver,kidney,pituitary, heart,brain,spleen and testis.Endocrinology 95:897
Oppenheimer,J.H.,Schwartz,H.L.,Shapiro,H.C. and Bersein,G.and Surks,M.I. 1970 Differences in primary cellular factors

influencing the metabolism and distribution of 3,3,3' L-triiodothyronine and L-thyroxine J Clin Invest 49:1016
Oppenheimer,J.H.,Schwartz,H.L.,Surks,M.I. 1972 Propylthioiuracil inhibits the conversion of L-thyroxine to L-triiodothyronine.An explanation of the antithyroxine effect of propylthiouracil and evidence supporting the concept that triiodothyronine is the active thyroid hormone.J.Clin.Invest 51:2493
Oppenheimer,J.H.,Schwartz,H.L.,Kaiser,F.E. and Mariash,C.N. 1981 A non-dialyzable factor in sera of patients with non-thyroidal illness inhibits binding of iodothyronines by charcoal,plasma proteins and cells,57th American Thyroid Assn.Meeting minneapolis Minn.T-10
Pearson,J.D.,Veall,N.,and Vetter,H. 1958 A practical method for plasma albumin turnover studies Strahlentherapie (Sonderb) 38:290
Pliam,N.B. and Goldfine,J.D. 1977 High affinity thyroid hormone binding sites on purified rat liver plasma membranes.Biochem.Biophys.Res.Comm.79:166
Pardrige ,W.M.,Slag,M.F.,Morley,J.E.,Elson,M.K.,Shafer,R.B. and Mietus,L.J. 1981 Hepatic bioavailability of serum thyroid hormones in non-thyroidal illness.J.Clin Endocrinol.Metab 53:913
Pardrige,W.M. 1981 Transport of protein-bound hormones into tissues in vivo.Endocrine Reviews 2:103
Rao,G.S.,Eckel,J.,Rao,M.L.and Breur,H. 1976 Uptake of thyroid hormone by isolated rat liver cells Biochem Biophys Res Comm 73:98
Rao,G.S. 1981 Mode of entry of steroid and thyroid hormones into cells.Mol.Cell Endocrinology 21:97
Samuels ,H.H.,J.Tsai and J. Casanova 1974 Thyroid hormone action:in vitro demonstration of putative receptors in isolated nuclei and soluble nuclear extracts.Science (Wash. D.C.),184:1188
Silva,J.E. 1972 Disposal rates of thyroxine and triiodothyronine in iodine-deficient rats.Endocrinology 91:1430
Silva,J.E.,Larsen,P.R. 1977 Pituitary nuclear 3,5,3'-triiodothyronine and thyrotropin secretion:an explanation for the effect of thyroxine.Science 198:617
Silva,J.E.,Dick,T.E. and Larsen,P.R. 1978 The contribution of local tissue thyroxine monodeiodination to the nuclear 3,5,3'-triiodothyronine in pituitary,liver and kidney of euthyroid rats.Endocrinology 103:1196
Schadlow,A.R.,Surks,M.I.,Schwartz,H.L.and Oppenheimer,J.H. 1972 Specific triiodothyronine binding sites in the anterior pituitary of the rat.Science 176:1252

Silva,J.E.,Kaplan,M.M.,Cheron,R.G.,Dick,T.E.,and Larsen,P.R. 1978 Thyroxine to 3,5,3-triiodothyronine conversion by rat anterior pituiatry and liver.Metabolism 27:1601

Silva,J.E., Differrential effect of the thyroid status on iodothyronine 5'-deiodinase activity and various enzymes of neonatal rat cerebral cortex (manuscript in preparation)

Silva,J.E.,Leonard,J.L.,Crantz,F.R. and Larsen,P.R. Evidence for two tissue-specific pathways for in vivo thyroxine 5'-deiodination in the rat J Clin.Invest.(in press)

Surks,M.I.,Oppenheimer,J.H. 1977 Concentration of L-thyroxine and L-triiodothyronine specifically bound to nuclear receptors in rat liver and kidney:quantitative evidence favoring a major role of T_3 in thyroid hormone action J.Clin.Invest.60:555

Tata,J.R.and Widnell,C.C. 1966 Ribonucleic acid synthesis during the early action of thyroid hormones Biochem.J. 98:604

Tommaselli,A.,Gravina,E.,and Roche,J. 1965 Physiological disposition of thyroid hormones in the heart of the rat Localization of the sino-ventricular conduction system In current topics in Thyroid Research C.Cassano and M. Andreoli,Editors Academic Press,New York,page 382

Visser,T.J.,Leonard,J.L.,Kaplan,M.M.and Larsen,P.R. 1981 Different pathways of iodothyronine 5'-deiodination in rat cerebral cortex.Biochem.Biophys.Res.Commun.101:1297

Volpert,E.M.,Grindberg,R.and Werner,S.C. 1962 Studies with mouse pituitary thyrotropic tumors.IV.Presence of 3,5,3'-triiodothyronine in certain mouse pituitary tumors after the injection of labelled L-thyroxine.Endocrinology 71:361

New Concepts in Thyroid Disease, pages 45–56

BIOCHEMICAL AND BIOPHYSICAL STUDIES ON THE ACTION OF THYROID HORMONES UPON CELL MEMBRANES

J.M. Pasquini*, T. De Paoli**, A.A. Hager**, P.I. Oteiza* and E.F. Soto*
*Depto. de Química Biológica and **Depto. de Físico Matemáticas, Fac. Farmacia y Bioquímica, UNBA, Junín 956, Buenos Aires, Argentina

INTRODUCTION

In the last few years we have studied the biosynthesis of phosphatidylcholine by brain and liver subcellular fractions and we have shown that mitochondria can synthesize part of their own membrane phospholipids, similarly to what occurs with the microsomal fraction (Soto et al., 1972; Krawiec et al., 1975).

In 1965, Nelson and Cornatzer published results demonstrating that the administration of L-thyroxine for six days to young adult rats resulted in changes in the incorporation of ^{32}P into different phospholipids of liver mitochondria. These results, as well as those reported by Sterling et al. (1977) seemed to indicate a possible direct effect of L-thyroxine upon mitochondria.

Recent experiments in our laboratories appear to support this point of view. We have shown that liver mitochondria isolated from thyroxine treated young rats showed a 50% decrease in the incorporation of labeled CDP-choline into phosphatidyl choline while no changes were observed in the microsomal fraction (Pasquini et al., 1980). Similar results were obtained with mitochondria and microsomal fraction isolated from the brains of 20 day old rats treated with thyroxine since birth (Faryna de Raveglia et al., 1982), demonstrating once more that, as previously stated by several investigators, the effect of thyroxine upon the nervous tissue depends on the age of the animal (Cocks et al., 1970; Pasquini et al., 1967).

References in the literature regarding the action of thyroid hormones upon the metabolism of cell membrane phospholipids are scarce and very little is known with reference to the final mechanism of action of this hormone. In order to obtain further information regarding the effects of thyroid hormones upon different subcellular membranes, as well as the molecular basis of some of the phenomena described in our laboratories, we decided to investigate the action of these hormones and some active and inactive analogs on phosphatidylcholine synthesis by liver mitochondria and microsomal fraction as well as their effect upon membrane conformation and structure using Electronic Spin Resonance (ESR) and Quenching of Intrinsic Fluorescence (QF).

EXPERIMENTAL PROCEDURES

Young adult Wistar rats of either sex were used in all the experiments. Livers were homogenized at 10% (w/v) in ice cold 0.32 M sucrose pH 7.4 using a Potter Elvehjem type homogenizer. The separation of subcellular fractions was done as previously described (Soto et al., 1972). Isolated liver mitochondria and microsomes were used to explore the "in vitro" action of L-thyroxine and of different analogs, upon the incorporation into phosphatidylcholine of radioactive CDP-choline, as well as for ESR and QF experiments.

Incubation Conditions

For the study of the incorporation of CDP-choline, the medium contained 37.5 mM. Tris-HCl buffer, pH 7.4; 10 mM. cysteine hydrochloride (adjusted to pH 7.4 with 0.1 M NaOH); 20 mM. $MgCl_2$; 0.17 M. sucrose; CDP-choline (0.10 µCi, 0.8 µmol) (final volume 2 ml) as described by Mc Murray and Dawson (1969).

The amount of liver fraction added to the incubation medium was equivalent to 50 mg fresh tissue of microsomal fraction and to 100 mg of fresh tissue of mitochondria per tube.

The fractions were first preincubated for 15 min. in the presence of different concentrations of added L-thyroxine or analogs and the reaction started by the addition of the complete medium. The incubations were carried out at 37°C for 30 minutes with continuous shaking. The incorporation of label was stopped by addition of chloroform:methanol 1:1

(v/v). Appropiate normal controls were processed similarly in all cases.

Lipid Extraction and Radioactive Counting

Extraction of lipids from the various samples and washing of the extracts was done according to Mc Murray and Dawson (1969). Radioactive counting was carried out in portions of the washed total lipid extracts evaporated to dryness in counting vials and redissolved in 10 ml of scintillation solution containing 4 gr of 2.5 diphenyloxazole and 0.1 gr of 1,4 bis (5 phenyloxazol 2 yl) benzene/litre of toluene. To check that the radioactivity was incorporated into phosphatidylcholine, lipids were separated by thin layer chromatography (TLC) as previously described (Seminario *et al.*, 1965) and the different areas of silica gel were scrapped off the plate and placed in counting vials containing 10 ml of scintillation solution.

Electron Spin Resonance (ESR)

Stearic acid labeled on C 16 with a paramagnetic radical (2-(14 carboxytetradecyl)-2-ethyl-4,4-dimethyl-3-oxazolidinyloxy) (16 D), (Syva Co. Palo Alto, California) was introduced into the mitochondrial membranes by incubation of an aliquot of mitochondria resuspended in 37.5 mM. Tris buffer pH 7.4, 2 mM. NaOH with an ethanolic solution of 16 D at 37°C for 15 minutes.

The ratio of labeled 16 D to mitochondrial protein was approximately 5-10 μg of 16 D per mg protein and the total amount of added ethanol was less than 1% (v/v). The sample was then placed in the cuvette for liquids and the ESR spectra were obtained using a Varian Spectrometer at 9 GHz and at room temperature (25°C), both in the presence and absence of thyroid hormones or analogs (see below). Quantitative evaluation of ESR spectra was carried out measuring time average parameters $T'_{//}$, $T'_{\perp}$, the parameter of order S and Δ 1 (Lowfield Linewidth) (Gaffney and Mc Namee, 1974).

Quenching of Intrinsic Fluorescence (QF).

A typical experiment was carried out as follows: To 3 ml of mitochondrial suspension in Tris buffer pH 7.4 (0.2-0.3 mg of protein/ml) were added 30 μl of ethanolic solution of 16 D in aliquots of 2 μl at the beginning of the experiment and 5 μl thereafter. Fluorescence was measured inmediately after the addition of each aliquot, using an Aminco Bowman Spectrophotofluorometer at room temperature (25°C). The intrinsic fluorescence of the membrane proteins was recorded as the total spectrum above 350 nm, excitation at 290 nm, slit width 1 mm. A similar set up was used to measure the effect of thyroid hormones at different concentrations (100 μl of hormone solution in Tris buffer pH 7.4, 2 mM NaOH), the hormone being added to the reaction cuvette prior to the addition of the spin label. $Fo/\Delta F = f(1/(N))$ was plotted and a straight line, which follows Stern-Volmer law (modified) was obtained (Lerher , 1971).

RESULTS

Table I shows the results of the "in vitro" incorporation of labeled CDP-choline into phosphatidylcholine of liver mitochondria in the presence and absence of thyroid hormones or analogs. L-thyroxine (L-T_4), at a concentration of 10^{-2}M.-10^{-5}M., decreased the incorporation of label to 40-50% of the control values, while at lower concentrations (10^{-7}M.-10^{-11}M.) the incorporation decreased to 60-65% of controls. D-thyroxine (D-T_4) showed no effect while L-triiodothyronine (L-T_3), triiodothyroacetic acid (TRIAC) and triiodopropionic acid (TP_3) decreased the incorporation only when concentrations as high as 10^{-3}M. were used. Tetraiodopropionic acid (TP_4), reversed triiodothyronine (r -T_3), monoiodotyrosine (MIT) and diiodotyrosine (DIT) tested at various concentrations had no effect.

A typical ESR spectrum obtained from normal liver mitochondria, labeled with 16 D, as well as the different parameters measured, is shown in Fig. 1A. Figure 1B shows the ESR spectrum obtained with a similar preparation to which T_4 was added. Analysis of these spectra indicated that no significant changes occurred in the parameters of order S, $T'_{//}$ or $T'_{\perp}$ while quite significant differences were found in Δ 1 (Lowfield Linewidth) even when very low concentration of L-T_4 (10^{-9}M.) were added to the medium. The results obtained measuring the above mentioned parameters in the presence of L-T_4, L-T_3 and some of the tested analogs (Table II) show that changes in Δ 1 are obtained only with L-T_4 and L-T_3.

Table I - Radioactive CDP-choline incorporation into phosphatidylcholine in the presence of thyroid hormones and different analogs.

	10^{-2}M	10^{-3}M	10^{-4}M	10^{-5}M	10^{-7}M	10^{-9}M	10^{-11}M
L-Thyroxine	40-50%	40-50%	-	40-50%	60%	65%	65%
	P 0.02	P 0.02		P 0.02	P 0.05	P 0.02	P 0.02
D-Thyroxine	-	105%	-	112%	108%	116%	109%
L-Triiodotironine	-	50%	-	95%	104%	-	-
		P 0.02					
Reverse triiodo-tironine	-	103%	-	101%	108%	-	-
Triiodo tiroacetic acid	-	20%	95%	111%	113%	-	-
		P 0.05					
Tetraiodo propionic acid	-	90%	-	103%	90%	-	-
Triiodopropionic acid	-	46%	-	95%	103%	-	-
		P 0.05					
Monoiodotyrosine	-	-	97%	114%	116%	-	-
Diiodotyrosine	-	-	113%	103%	96%	-	-

Incubation conditions are described under Experimental Procedures. The enzymatic activity is expressed as percent of a control, taken as 100%.

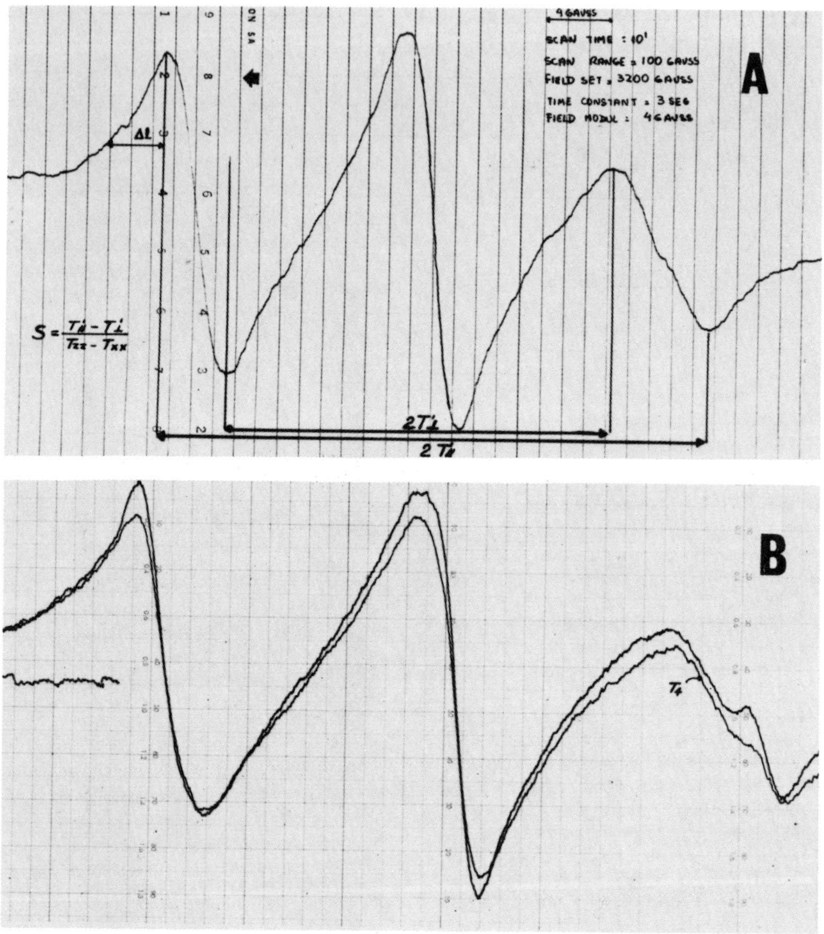

Figure 1. ESR spectra obtained from mitochondria. A= shows the parameters measured (for details see text). B= typical spectrum with and without the addition of L-thyroxine.

Table II - Changes in the Δ 1 (Lowfield Linewidth) obtained in the presence of thyroid hormones and different analogs.

	CONCENTRATION	
	5×10^{-7}M	5×10^{-9}M
L-thyroxine	24.0 ± 2.0	24.0 ± 2.0
L-triiodotironine	18.2 ± 2.0	18.0 ± 2.0
D-thyroxine	N.S.	N.S.
Triiodotiroacetic acid	N.S.	N.S.
Monoiodotirosine	N.S.	N.S.
Diiodotirosine	N.S.	N.S.

Results are expressed as percent of change in Δ 1.
N.S. = non significant.

Since it was difficult to accept that L-T_4 (or L-T_3) could act directly upon membrane phospholipids in mitochondria, we decided to investigate possible modifications induced by this hormone at the protein-lipid interphase, studying quenching of fluorescence of the tryptophane groups, produced by 16 D used as a probe (Fig. 2).

The figure represents the results obtained when Fo/Δ F is plotted as a function of the concentration of 16 D. It can be seen that quenching constant Kq for a preparation of mitochondria in the absence of L-T_4 or L-T_3 was 5.4×10^3 (M^{-1}) while in the presence of either hormone at a concentration of 8.3×10^{-8}M., the value of Kq dropped to 1.3×10^4 (M^{-1}) indicating that a marked change in the quenching of fluorescence produced by 16 D occurred when these hormones were present in the medium.

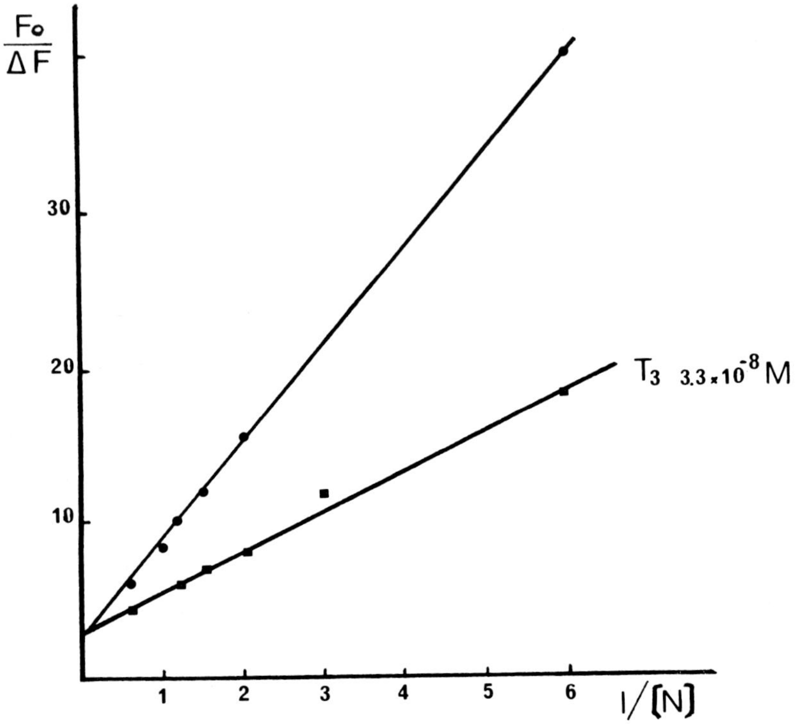

Figure 2. Modified Stern-Volmer plots of the quenching of the intrinsic fluorescence in mitochondrial membrane by stearic acid nitroxide spin label in the presence and absence of L-T_3. Fo: initial fluorescence; Δ F: change in fluorescence due to addition of the quencher at a concentration (N).

DISCUSSION

Enzymes participating in the synthesis of phospholipids were first described by Wilgram and Kennedy (1963) as endoplasmic reticulum enzymes. Work by Mc Caman and Cook (1966), Stoffel and Schieffer (1968), Kaiser (1969) and more recently by Van Schijndel et al. (1973) however, suggested that brain and liver mitochondria were able to synthesize phospholipids through the CTP mediated pathway. In previous papers we have dealt extensively with this controversial subject and have come to the conclusion that mitochondria can synthesize at least part of their own phospholipids (Soto et al., 1977). Moreover we have shown that the synthesis of phosphatidylcholine by mitochondria could be influenced by L-thyroxine (Pasquini et al., 1980). A study of the possible mechanisms through which this hormone exerts its action upon the synthesis of this phospholipid at the mitochondrial level were the object of the studies reported in this communication.

The concept that thyroid hormones act directly upon cell organelles different from the nucleus, contradict evidences showing that one of their first effects is to increase genetic transcription. The interactions of thyroid hormones with mitochondria have been extensively studied, but the concentrations of hormones necessary to obtain effects were much higher that those observed under physiological conditions.

In all our experiments, both "in vivo" and "in vitro", the effects of the hormone upon phosphatidyl choline biosynthesis in mitochondria were obtained at very low concentrations. These facts would give support to the idea of studying the effects of thyroid hormones upon the activity of membrane bound enzymes as a useful tool for the investigation of physiological and biochemical perturbations produced by hypo or hyperthyroidism.

The apparently high stereospecificity of mitochondrial "receptor/s" could be of physiological importance, since according to our results, the effect of thyroid hormones upon the incorporation of CDP-choline into mitochondrial phosphatidylcholine depends on the following structural requirements: 1) L-alanine side chain, since analogs in which it is replaced by acetate or propionate are inactive. 2) L-configuration since D-thyroxine has no effect. 3) Diphenyl ether structure, since MIT and DIT have no activity and 4) the four positions (3,5,3' and 5') should be substituted, since L-T_3 and r-T_3 are inactive.

The results of ESR and QF experiments indicate quite clearly that thyroid hormones produce an action upon mitochondrial membranes which in turn could alter the activity of the enzyme responsible for the incorporation of CDP-choline into phosphatidylcholine (i.e.: 1,2 diglyceride CDP-choline choline phosphotransferase), an enzyme closely related to membranes.

The maximal distance between tryptophane (tyrosin) and

nitroxide groups should not exceed 5-6 A° and the nitroxide radical used as a probe, must be lying inmersed in the hydrophobic portion of the lipid bylayer of the membrane (Marsh and Barrantes, 1978). Since changes in the quenching constants of the aromatic groups interacting with the nitroxide radicals are detected, it seems reasonable to assume that a structural change or modification is taking place in some intrinsic protein (s) of the membrane, under the action of the hormone.

We have no clear explanation for the finding that L-T_4 affects the incorporation of CDP-choline in mitochondria without affecting it in the microsomal fraction. Hulbert et al. (1976) have shown that in rat liver mitochondria, membrane lipid insaturation increases, the temperature limits of the membrane phase transition decreases and the Ea of succinate oxidase increases after thyroidectomy. All these parameters change in the opposite direction only 12 hs after treatment with thyroxine, indicating that the actions of thyroid hormones on the mitochondrial membrane are very rapid. Experiments carried out in our laboratories (unpublished) have shown that Arrhenius plots of the enzymatic activity of mitochondrial CDP-choline, choline phosphotransferase indicate a phase transition at about 23°C, while similar plots obtained with microsomal membranes do not show a phase transition within the range of temperatures explored by us (10°C-40°C). It is possible that the phase transition temperature of microsomal membranes might be lower than the ones explored in our study.

The results of our ESR spectra and the quenching of intrinsic fluorescence do not agree completely with those obtained in the studies of incorporation of CDP-choline, since only L-T_4 produces changes in the latter experiments, while both L-T_4 and L-T_3 are effective in the former ones. One possible explanation for this discrepancy it that in the experiments mentioned in the text, we used stearic acid labeled in the C 16 position and that we could be measuring a perturbation in the membrane which does not occur at the specific binding site of 1,2 diglyceride: CDP-choline choline phosphotransferase. To explore this hypothesis we are presently carrying out experiments using fatty acids labeled in two different positions of their hydrocarbon chain. On the other hand, it should be mentioned that De Mendoza and Farías (1978) have shown that L-T_3, L-T_4 and TSH appear to be involved in a particular type of interplay in the phenomenon of allosteric desensitization produced by L-T_3. Obviously, both actions have to be due to iodothyronines acting upon the membrane but affecting the enzyme studied in a completely opposite way.

Our results seem to support the hypothesis that thyroid hormones produce specific actions upon structure and function of mitochondria and that some of the quick physiological effects of these hormones might be due to this interaction. Further work is needed in order to validate this hypothesis.

REFERENCES

Cocks JA, Balazs R, Johnson AL, Eayrs JT (1970) Effects of thyroid hormone on the biochemical maturation of rat brain: conversion of glucose-carbon into aminoacids. J. Neurochem. 17: 1275-1285.

De Mendoza D, Farías RN (1978) Effect of cold exposure on rat erythrocyte membrane-bound acetylcholinesterase. J. Biol. Chem. 253: 6249-6254.

Faryna de Raveglia IA, Pasquini JM, Soto EF (1982) Effect of thyroid disfunction upon phospholipid composition and CDP-choline incorporation in mitochondria and microsomal fraction isolated from liver and brain of suckling rats. Neuroch. Res. 7: 1377-1387.

Gaffney BJ, Mc Namee CM (1974) Spin label measurements in membrane. In Methods in Enzymology 32 (B): 161-198.

Hulbert AJ, Augee ML, Raison JK (1976) The influence of thyroid hormones on the structure and function of mitochondrial membranes. Biochimica Biophys. Acta 455: 597-601.

Kaiser W (1969) Incorporation of phospholipid precursors into isolated rat liver mitochondria. Eur. J. Biochem. 8: 120-127.

Krawiec L, Pasquini JM, Soto EF (1975) Incorporation of CDP-choline (Methyl-^{14}C) into lecithin of adult rat liver mitochondria and microsomes. Acta Physiol. Latino Americana XXV: 69-76.

Lerher SS (1971) Solute perturbation of protein fluorescence. The quenching of the tryptophyl fluorescence of model compounds and of lysozyme by iodide ion. Biochemistry 10: 3254-3263.

Marsh D, Barrantes FJ (1978) Immobilized lipid in acetylcholine receptor-rich membranes from Torpedo marmorate. Proc. Natl. Acad. Sci USA 75: 4329-4333.

Mc Caman RE, Cook K (1966) Intermediary metabolism of phospholipids in brain tissue. J. Biol. Chem. 241: 3390-3394.
Mc Murray WC, Dawson RMC (1969) Phospholipid exchange reactions within the liver cell. Biochem. J. 112: 91-108.
Nelson DR, Cornatzer WE (1965) Role of the thyroid in the synthesis of heart, liver and kidney mitochondrial phospholipids. Endocrinology 77: 37-44.
Pasquini JM, Kaplun B, García Argiz CA, Gómez CJ (1967) Hormonal regulation of brain development. I. Effect of neonatal thyroidectomy upon nucleic acids proteins and two enzymes in developing cerebral cortex and cerebellum of the rat. Brain Res. 6: 621-643.
Seminario L, Soto EF, Cohan T (1965) Quantitative analysis of phospholipids by thin layer chromatography. J. Chromat. 17: 513-519.
Soto EF, Pasquini JM, Krawiec L (1972) In vitro incorporation of (^3H) methyl choline into phosphatidylcholine of rat liver subcellular fractions. Archs. Biochem. Biophys. 150: 362-370.
Soto EF, Najle R, Raveglia IAF de, Pasquini JM (1977) Metabolism of phosphatidylcholine in the Central Nervous System. In Bazán N, Brenner RP, Giusto NM (eds): "Function and Biosynthesis of Lipids", New York, Plenum Press, p 345-360.
Sterling K, Lazarus JH, Milch PO, Sakurada T, Brenner MA (1978) Mitochondrial thyroid hormone receptor. Localization and physiological significance. Science 20: 1126-1129.
Stoffel W, Schiefer HG (1968) Biosynthesis and composition of phosphatides in outer and inner mitochondrial membranes. Hoppe Seyler's Z Physiol. Chem. 349: 1017-1026.
Van Schijndel BC, Reitsema A, Scherphof GL (1973) In vitro stimulation of lecithin synthesis in rat liver mitochondria and microsomes after treatment with phospholipase C. Biochem. Biophys. Res. Commun. 55: 568-573.
Wilgram GF, Kennedy EP (1963) Intracellular distribution of some enzymes catalyzing reactions in the biosynthesis of complex lipids. J. Biol. Chem. 238: 2615-2619.

New Concepts in Thyroid Disease, pages 57–73

METABOLIC AND ULTRASTRUCTURAL EFFECTS OF HYPOTHYROIDISM UPON ENDOCRINE PANCREAS

Gagliardino,J.J.; Cortizo,Ana María; Pisarev,M.A.; Chazenbalk,G.D. and Gómez Dumm, C.L. with the technical assistance of Elma E.P. de Gagliardino.
CENEXA-Centro de Endocrinología Experimental y Aplicada(UNLP-CONICET);Instituto de Embriología,Biología e Histología,Facultad de Ciencias Médicas,UNLP, 60 y 120, 1900 La Plata and Division Bioquímica Nuclear, Comisión Nacional de Energía Atómica, ARGENTINA.

The relationship between thyroid hormones and the function of the endocrine pancreas has been already demonstrated both at the clinical and experimental level(Houssay(1944);Malaisse et al.(1967); Katsilambros et al.(1972);Marecek and Feldman (1973);Shah and Cerchio(1973);Renauld et al.(1974); Lenzen et al.(1975);Renauld et al.(1975);Lenzen et al.(1976);Lenzen et al.(1976);Zamrazil et al(1976); Andersen et al.(1977);Lenzen(1978);Lenzen and Klöppel(1978);Ahrén and Lundquist(1981).There is a general agreement about the lower B cell capacity to release insulin observed in the hypothyroid state(Malaisse et al.(1967);Katsilambros et al. (1972);Shah and Cerchio(1973);Renauld et al.(1974); Lenzen et al.(1976);Zamrazil et al.(1976);Ahrén and Lundquist(1981).Conversely,controversial results have been published regarding the effect of hyperfunction of the thyroid gland on insulin secretion(Marecek and Feldman(1973);Lenzen et al. (1975);Andersen et al.(1977);Ahrén and Lundquist (1981).

Despite the large number of experiments performed regarding the effect of thyroid hormones on the secretory function of pancreatic islets, neither the metabolic nor the ultrastructural substract for such effect has been demonstrated at the islets level. Furthermore, whether this effect is exerted by the thyroid hormone directly on the islets or is simply the consequence of the general metabolic disturbance induced by the hypo or hyperthyroid state, is still an open question.

In the present report, using isolated islets from normal and hypothyroid rats, we have studied the relationship between glucose-induced insulin secretion and the glucose oxidation and calcium uptake by the islets, as well as their ultrastructural aspects. Furthermore, the ability of normal islets to deiodinate 125-I-T_4 was also studied.

MATERIAL AND METHODS

Chemicals: Collagenase was obtained from Serva Feinbiochemica. Heidelberg; Trasylol(R) (100.000 KIU) was kindly provided by Bayer Argentina; {U-^{14}C} glucose (3.0 mCi/nmol); ^{45}Ca (5.7 µCi/ml) as {$^{45}CaCl_2$} and Thyroxine L-(^{125}I)-(100-150 µCi/µg) from New England Nuclear, Boston, Mass; bovine albumin (fraction V) and other reagents of the purest available grade were from Sigma Chemical Co, St. Louis, Mo. Guinea Pig anti insulin serum was kindly provided by Dr. Raúl Gutman.

Animals and preparation of islets: Wistar male rats about 100 g b.w. were used. Half of them were rendered hypothyroid (H) by administration of a single intraperitoneal injection of 700µCi ^{131}I in saline solution, while the remaining animals were used as controls (C). The experiments were performed at least 5 weeks after the iodine injection. Thyroid function was assessed by individual body weight control and the circulating levels of T_3 and T_4 (RIA kit, Diagnostic Products Corporation, Los Angeles, Ca.)

Pancreases from control of hypothyroid rats were used to obtain isolated islets by collagenase digestion (Lacy and Kostianovsky (1967).

Insulin secretion: Groups of 5 islets were incubated for 60 min at 37°C in 0.6 ml Krebs Ringer Bicarbonate (KRB buffer), pH 7.4 with 1% bovine serum albumin (BSA), the protease inhibitor (Trasylol(R)), and glucose 3.3 or 16.6 mM.The preparation was previously gassed with a mixture of 95% O_2:5% CO_2 (Gagliardino et al(1974).Aliquots from the media were separated for insulin determination(Herbert et al.(1965).

Glucose oxidation:Batches of 20 islets were incubated for 2 h at 37°C in KRB buffer with{U-^{14}C} glucose(3.0 mCi/nmol) in the presence of either 3.3 or 16.6 mM glucose.The production of $^{14}CO_2$ was measured as described elsewhere(Ashcroft et.al. (1970).

^{45}Ca uptake:Groups of 100 islets were incubated in 300 μl of KRB with 1% BSA,glucose 3.3 or 16.6 mM and ^{45}Ca(20 μCi)for 90 min at 37°C.At the end of the incubation period,the incubation medium was removed and replaced by a medium of identical composition but without ^{45}Ca.After five succesive washes,the islets were individually transferred,in groups of 10,to a scintillation vial for radioactive determination(Malaisse-Lagae and Malaisse(1971).

Electron microscopy: Four pancreases of each group of rats,immersed in phosphate buffered p-formaldehyde-glutaraldehyde solution(Karnovsky (1965),were dissected under a stereo microscope. The islets obtained were fixed in the same buffer-osmium tetroxide and embedded in araldite. Ultrathin sections were mounted on copper grids,stained with uranyl acetate and lead citrate and examined with a Siemens Elmiskop I electron microscope.No less than 10 islets per animal were observed and more than 15 B cells in each islet were studied with different magnifications ranging from x 3.000 to x 40.000.

^{125}I-T_4 deiodination:Groups of 100 islets were incubated in the darkness at 37°C during 15 or 60 minutes,in 500 μl of Krebs Ringer Bicarbonate buffer pH 7.4,with the addition of glucose(3.3 or 16.6 mM)and ^{125}I-T_4(1μCi).

At the end of the incubation period,the islets were washed twice in fresh KRB buffer,resuspended in 200 μl of 1% propylthiouracil in 20 mM TRIS-buffer pH 7.7,sonicated for 10 seconds and finally extracted with ethanol.All these steps were performed in the darkness. Aliquots of these extracts were run in paper chromatography for identification of iodothyronines following the procedure described by Bellabarba et al.(1968).

Results are given as mean ± SEM for the number of observations in parentheses.The significance of differences was assessed by using the Student's t test.

RESULTS

Body weigth: body weight in control and ^{131}I injected animals was around 100 g at the beginning of the experiments.The later groups,however,showed a significantly lower growth-rate as shown in Fig. 1.In that figure,every point represents mean of 10 animals ± SEM.At the time of the experiments,body weight in control and hypothyroid animals was 245±4.3 g and 170±5.4 g respectively.

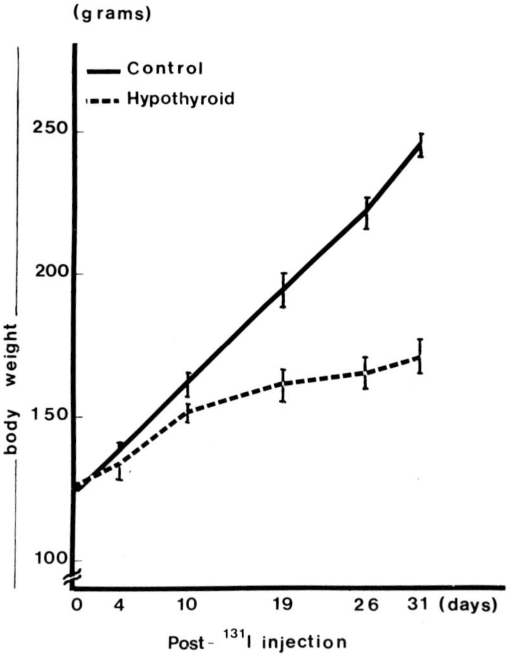

Figure 1

T_3 and T_4 circulating levels:serum thyroid hormone levels were determined in both groups of animals at the time of sacrifice. Table 1 shows that both T_3 and T_4 in hypothyroid animals were significantly lower than in control ($P<0.001$).

TABLE 1

GROUP	T_3 (ng/dl)	T_4 (µg/dl)
CONTROL	60.3 ± 4.30 (28)	2.45 ± 0.13 (28)
HYPOTHYROID	27.5 ± 2.95 (37)	0.65 ± 0.08 (37)
C vs H	P<0.001	P<0.001

Each value represents the mean ± SEM. Number of cases in parentheses. Significance is expressed as P value.

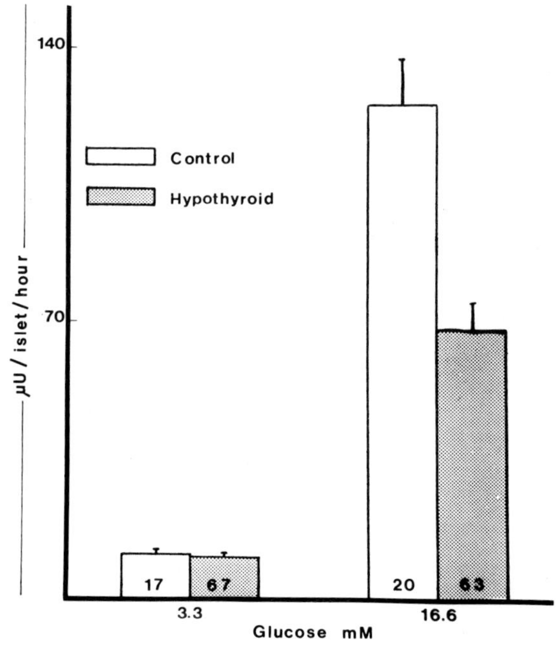

Figure 2

In Fig.2, insulin secretion (µU/islets/h) is represented in each group as the mean ± SEM. Number of cases is indicated within the corresponding bar. Insulin release significantly increased when glucose was raised in the medium from 3.3 to 16.6 mM. Insulin secretion was similar in both groups at low glucose concentration. However at 16.6 mM glucose, the response of hypothyroid islets was significanly lower than control islets($P<0.001$).

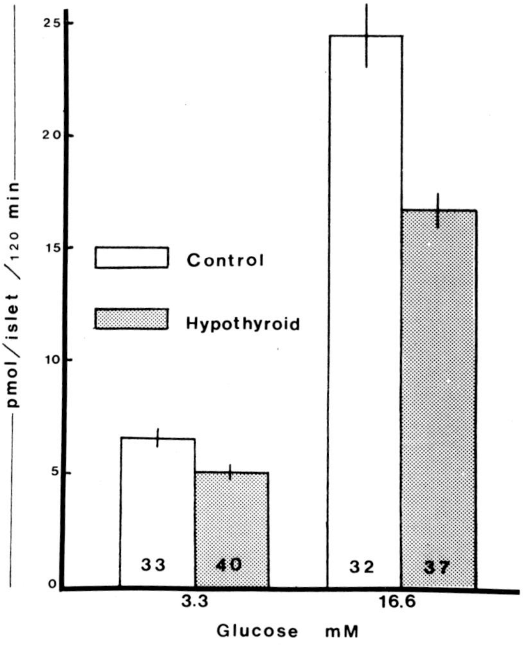

Figure 3

In Fig.3, glucose metabolism($^{14}CO_2$ production pmol/islet/2 h), is represented in each group as the mean ± SEM. Number of cases is indicated within the corresponding bar. $^{14}CO_2$ production from{$U^{14}C$} glucose depends, in both groups, on the glucose concentration in the medium, being significantly higher in the presence of 16.6 mM glucose. Again, $^{14}CO_2$ production was significantly lower in hypothyroid islets both in the presence of 3.3($P<0.02$) and 16.6 mM ($P<0.001$) glucose.

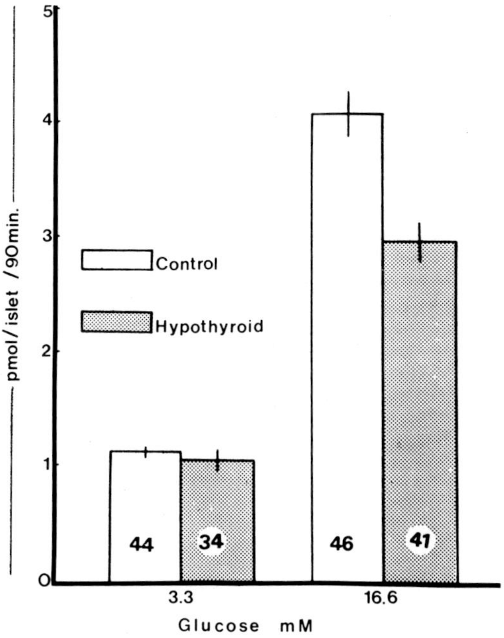

Figure 4

In Fig.4,calcium uptake(pmol/islet/90 min) is represented in each group as the mean ± SEM.Number of cases is indicated within the corresponding bar. $^{45}Ca^{2+}$ uptake showed the well known glucose concentration dependence.In this case,the uptake was similar in both groups in the presence of 3.3 mM glucose but significantly lower in hypothyroid islets($P<0.001$) at 16.6 mM glucose.

Ultrastructural results: the electron microscopic study of the islets revealed the four different cell types previously described in rat endocrine pancreas. However,only B cells presented clear changes between hypothyroid and control animals. These cells appeared with normal characteristics in islets from control rats(Fig.5).

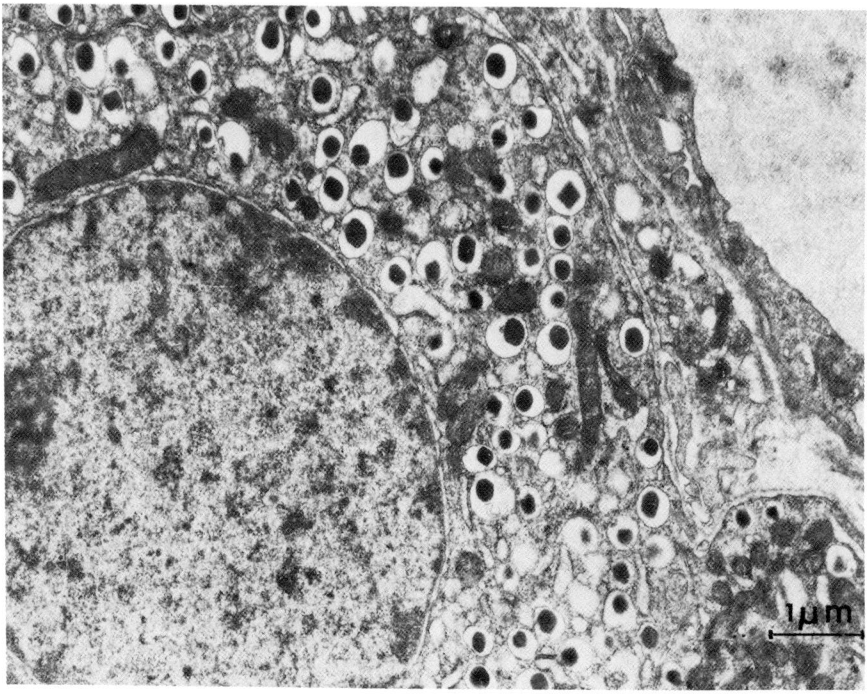

Figure 5. Electrommicrography of a normal B cell from a control rat.

On the other hand, many B cells of pancreases from hypothyroid animals(Fig.6) showed a large amount of secretory granules, most of them with a marked increase of the clear halo.Their dense cores were of normal or diminished size. Lucent vesicles which size was similar to that of the secretory granules, but lacking the dense core, were frequently found. These vesicles might be the result of sections that do not reach a small or excentrical dense core.

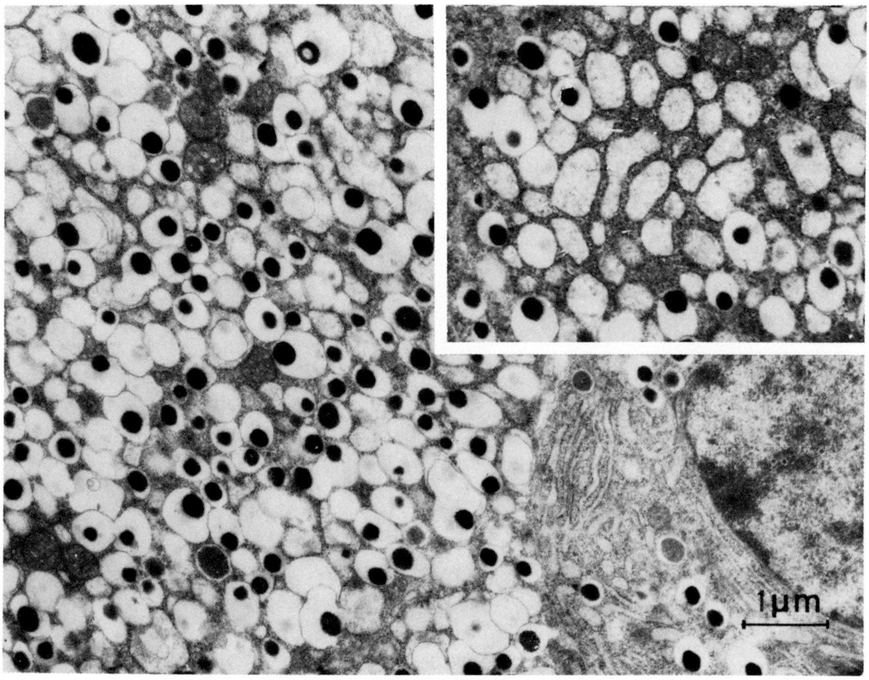

Figure 6. B cells from a H rat. Numerous secretory granules with an enlarged clear halo are observed. A number of vesicles contain a small dense core or appear empty. Notice the scarce cytoplasmic matrix comparing with the cell in the right lower corner, or with a normal B cell (Fig.5). Inset: dilated cisternae of granular endoplasmic reticulum.

In hypothyroid rats, the granular endoplasmic reticulum of B cells (Fig.6, inset) appeared frequently composed of dilated round or irregular cisternae containing a slightly dense material. The occurence of emiocytotic figures, pales granules and lysosomes did not reveal striking differences between the control and the hypothyroid group.

Deiodination of $^{125}I-T_4$: Table 2 shows the results of normal islets incubated with $^{125}I-T_4$ in the presence of low and high glucose concentration

TABLE 2

DEIODINATION OF $^{125}I-T_4$ BY ISOLATED ISLETS

Glucose (mM)	Percentage of total radioactivity in the chromatograms				
	ORIGIN	IODIDE	rT_3	T_4	T_3
3.3 60 min	3.45±0.01	7.08±0.18	2.48±0.04	72.33±4.01	3.83±0.08
16.6 60 min	3.88±0.06	12.21±0.93	4.82±0.93	62.76±1.78	5.79±0.38
16.6 15 min	3.20±0.26	7.76±0.22	4.67±0.40	68.87±3.07	6.24±0.56

Isolated islets were incubated with $^{125}I-T_4$ as described in methods. Values are expressed as mean ±SEM.

Origin between groups N.S.
Iodide 16.6 mM(60 min) vs 16.6 mM(15 min) $P<0.005$
16.6 mM(60 min) vs 3.3 mM(60 min) $P<0.005$
rT_3 16.6 mM(60 min) vs 16.6 mM(15 min) N.S.
16.6 mM(60 min) vs 3.3 mM(60 min) $P<0.05$
T_4 Between groups N.S.
T_3 16.6 mM(60 min) vs 16.6 mM(15 min) N.S.
16.6 mM(60 min) vs 3.3 mM(60 min) $P<0.005$

in the medium. T_4 was deiodinated by the islets to I^-, T_3 and rT_3. The production of T_3 and rT_3 depends on the glucose concentration in the medium, being significantly higher in the presence of 16.6 mM glucose.

The amount of T_3 and rT_3 produced by the islets incubated by either 15 or 60 minutes in the presence of 16.6 mM glucose was almost the same. However, the I^- production was significantly larger at 60 than at 15 minutes.

DISCUSSION

The changes in insulin secretion presently described in hypothyroid islets agree with data previously reported by other authors(Houssay(1944); Malaisse et al.(1967);Katsilambros et al.(1972); Shah and Cerchio(1973);Renauld et al.(1974);Lenzen et al.(1976);Zamrazil et al.(1976);Ahrén and Lundquist (1981).

According to our results, the modification in glucose-induced insulin release in hypothyroid islets can be ascribed to changes in B cell capacity to handle glucose and calcium. The changes observed at the ultrastructural level also lend further support to such assumption.

The relationship between glucose metabolism and insulin secretion in pancreatic islets has been previously demonstrated(Ashcroft et al.(1970);Ashcroft(1980). In our experiments, the amount of insulin released in control and hypothyroid islets group was tightly related to the corresponding B cell oxidizing capacity. Accordingly, glucose metabolism in the islets might be controlled, at least in part, by the circulating levels of thyroid hormones. This control of glucose metabolism at the B cell level, could explain the lower insulin secretion observed in hypothyroid islets.

The concentration of extracellular and intracellular calcium plays an important role in insulin secretion(Hellman(1975);Malaisse et al(1978). Moreover, calcium uptake has been shown to be related to extracellular glucose concentration and consequently to insulin secretion(Malaisse-Lagae and Malaisse(1971);Ashcroft(1980);Hellman(1975);Malaisse et al.(1978).

Calcium uptake was significantly decreased in the islets from hypothyroid rats.Hence,calcium uptake is another factor involved in the mechanism of thyroid hormones action on insulin secretion.

Although the changes in glucose metabolism could secondary affect calcium uptake,it might be possible that in the islets,like in other tissues (Wallach et al.(1972),thyroid hormones directly modify this parameter.

We have previously shown that glucose-induced insulin secretion was significantly affected by glucocorticoids and female steroid hormones(Borelli and Gagliardino(1979);García and Gagliardino(1980). This effect was tightly related to the changes produced on glucose and calcium handling by the islets. On account of such results and the ones presently reported,we could suggest that glucose and calcium metabolism in pancreatic islets are under hormonal control.Therefore,these metabolic changes could be the main path for the effect of several hormones on insulin secretion.

The B cell from hypothyroid animals showed a clear cut picture.In addition to the fact that the number of B granules was larger than that usually seen in normal islets,they were of abnormal characteristics,showing an enlarged clear space between the dense hormonal material and their membrane. Moreover,their rough endoplasmic reticulum was significantly enlarged suggesting an increased biosynthetic activity. Conversely,no signs of increased releasing activity were present in the hypothyroid B cell. This later ultrastructural aspect can be easily correlated with the diminished insulin release obtained <u>in vitro</u> by the isolated islets challenged with glucose. Hence,it seems to be that the hypothyroidism would produce an uncoupling effect between synthesis and secretion at the B cell level.

It is generally accepted that 3,5,3'-triiodothyronine(T_3)contributes in a major portion to the overall metabolic effects of the thyroid hormones at the peripheral level(Larsen et al.(1981);Chopra et al.(1978).It is also evident that most of the circulating T_3 in normal conditions arises,not by direct secretion from the thyroid gland,but rather from the peripheral monodeiodination of thyroxine (T_4) in its outer ring at the 5' position.

An alternate pathway of peripheral T_4 metabolism involves monodeiodination of T_4 in its inner ring to yield 3,3'5'-triiodothyronine(reverse T_3 or rT_3(Larsen et al.(1981);Chopra et al(1978). While T_3 is several times more potent than T_4,rT_3 appears to be hormonally inactive.Therefore,it is apparent that peripheral tissues are equipped with mechanisms that can act on T_4 to generate more potent as well as less potent iodothyronines compared to the parent compound.Accordingly,the predominant pathway leading peripherally to the generation of T_3 or rT_3 from T_4 might be an important metabolic control point with respect to thyroid hormone action.

In our experimental conditions,isolated islets were able to deiodinate T_4 both in its outer and inner ring with the consequent production of T_3 and rT_3 respectively. These two deiodination systems showed a clear glucose dependence,being both stimulated by the presence of high glucose concentration in the incubation medium.These results resemble those previously reported in liver tissue (Balsan and Ingbar(1978);Harris et al.(1978);Balsam and Ingbar(1979).In that case it was proved that T_3 formation was impaired in preparations of liver from fasted rats and this effect was prevented by in vivo glucose administration.However,in this experiments,the impaired T_3 production by fasted liver tissue was not overcome by rising the glucose concentration in the incubation medium(Balsam and Ingbar(1978);Harris et al.(1978);Balsam and Ingbar(1979).Therefore,our results would be the first demonstration of a deiodination process of T_4 by pancreatic islets being this tissue also the first one affected directly by glucose in vitro.

The effect of glucose upon the T_4 deiodination has been attributed to the NADPH provision throughout the hexosemonophosphate shunt(Balsam and Ingbar(1979).However,it has recently been suggested that the insulin molecule by itself might be the main stimulator for T_4 deiodination (Sato and Robbins(1981).Since the pentose pathway is very active in the islets and the insulin concentration within them is the highest achieved in the body,both explanations are compatible with our present results.

Similar percentages of T_3 and rT_3 were obtained in islets incubated for 15 or 60 minutes.However, the latter showed significantly higher levels of I^-.These results,would indicate that the islets are able to regulate both the relationship and the absolute intracellular levels of active and inactive iodothyronines.The presence of such fine mechanism strongly argue in favor of a local action of thyroid hormones on pancreatic islets.

On account of our results we could suggest that hypothyroidism in the rat is followed by a decreased B cell capacity to release insulin.This effect might be due to a defect in the B cell efficiency to handle glucose and calcium. This impaired function is also supported by an altered ultrastructural picture of the B cells.Furthermore,the selective deiodination of T_4 by normal islets, strongly suggest a possible direct effect of thyroid hormones on endocrine pancreas.

ACKNOWLEDGEMENTS

The authors wish to thank Mrs.Ana Galeano and Mrs.Susana Rivas for technicasl assistance and Miss Silvia Lunati for careful typing.

This project was partially supported by grants from CONICET,CIC,Pcia. de Bs.As. and SECYT of Argentina.

A.M.Cortizo is fellow from CIC,Pcia.de Bs.As.; G.D.Chazenbalk is fellow from CONICET;C.L.Gómez Dumm is member from the Carrera del Investigador, CIC,Pcia. de Bs.As.;M.A.Pisarev and J.J.Gagliardino are members from the Carrera del Investigador, CONICET and E.E.P.de Gagliardino is member from Carrera del Personal de Apoyo,CONICET.

REFERENCES

Ahrén B ,Lundquist I (1981).Insulin secretory response to different secretagogues in hyper and hypothyroid mice.Acta Endocrinol 97:508.

Andersen O O,FriisTh,Ottensen D(1977).Glucose

tolerance and insulin secretion in hypothyroidism. Acta Endocrinol 84:561.

Ashcroft S J H(1980).Glucoreceptor mechanism and the control of insulin release and biosynthesis.Diabetologia 18:5.

Ashcroft S J H,Hedeskov C J,Randle P J(1970). Glucose metabolism in mouse pancreatic islets. Biochem J 118:143.

Balsam A,Ingbar S H(1978).The influence of fasting,diabetes and several pharmacological agents on the pathways of thyroxine metabolism in rat liver.J Clin Invest 62:415.

Balsam A,Ingbar S H(1979).Observations on the factors that control the generation of triiodothyronine from thyroxine in rat liver and the nature of the defect induced by fasting.J Clin Invest 63: 1145.

Bellabarba D,Peterson R E,Sterling K(1968).An improved method for chromatography of iodotironines. J Clin Endcrinol & Metab 28:305.

Borelli M I,Gagliardino J J(1979).Effects of glucocorticoids on glucose metabolism and insulin secretion in pancreatic islets.IRCS,Medical Sci 7: 468.

Chopra I J,Solomon D H,Chopra U,Wu S Y,Fischer D A(1978).Pathways of metabolism of thyroid hormones.Rec Prog Horm Res 34:521.

Gagliardino J J,Nierle C,Pfeiffer E F(1974). The effect of serotonin on in vitro insulin secretion and biosynthesis in mice.Diabetologia 10:411.

García M E,Gagliardino J J(1980).Effects of estrogen and progesterone upon insulin secretion and glucose metabolism in pancreatic islets.IRCS, Medical Sci 8:448.

Harris A R C,Fang S L,Vegenakis A G,Braverman L E(1978).Effect of starvation,nutriment replacement,and hypothyroidism on in vitro hepatic T_4 to T_3 conversion in the rat.Metabolism 27:1680.

Hellman B(1975).The significance of calcium for glucose stimulation of insulin release.Endocrinol 97:392.

Herbert V,Lau K S,Gottlieb Ch W,Bleicher S J (1965).Coated-charcoal immunoassay of insulin.J Clin Endocr 25:1375.

Houssay B A(1944).Thyroid and metathyroid diabetes.Endocrinol 35:158.

Karnovsky J M(1965).A formaldehyde-glutaraldehyde fixative of high osmolarity for use in electron microscopy.J Cell Biol 27:137(A).

Katsilambros N,Ziegler R,Schatz H,Hinz M,Maier V,Pfeiffer E F(1972).Intravenous glucose tolerance and insulin secretion in the rat after thyroidectomy.Horm Metab Res 4:377.

Lacy P,Kostianovsky M(1967).Method for the isolation of intact islets of Langerhans from the rat pancreas.Diabetes 16:35.

Larsen P R,Silva J E,Kaplan M M(1981).Relationship between circulating and intracellular thyroid hormones:physiological clinical implications. Endocrine Rev 2:87.

Lenzen S(1978).Dose-response studies on the inhibitory effect of thyroid hormones on insulin secretion.Metabolism 27:81.

Lenzen S,Jost H G,Hasselblatt A(1976).The inhibition of insulin secretion for the perfused rat pancreas after thyroxine treatment.Diabetologia 12: 495.

Lenzen S,Jost H G,Hasselblatt A(1976).Thyroid function and insulin secretion from the perfused pancreas in the rat.Endocrinology 99:125.

Lenzen S,Klöppel G(1978).Insulin secretion and the morphological and metabolis characteristics of pancreatic islets of hyperthyroid ob/ob mice. Endocrinol 103:1546.

Lenzen S,Panten U,Hasselblatt A(1975).Thyroxine treatment and insulin secretion in the rat. Diabetologia 11:49.

Malaisse W J,Herchuelz A,Devis G,Somers G,Boschero A C,Hutton J C,Kawazy S,Sener A,Atwater I J, Duncan G,Ribaler B,Rojas E(1978).Regulation of calcium fluxes and their regulatory roles in pancreatic islets.Ann N Y Acad Sci U S A.307:562.

Malaisse-Lagae F,Malaisse W J(1971).Stimulus-secretion coupling of glucose-induced insulin release.III Uptake of ^{45}calcium by isolated islets of Langerhans.Endocrinology 88:72.

Malaisse W J,Malaisse-Lagae F,Mc Craw E F (1967).Effects of thyroid function upon insulin secretion.Diabetes 16:643.

Marecek R L,Feldman J M(1973).Effect of hyperthyroidism on insulin and glucose dynamics in rabbits.Endocrinology 92:1304.

Renauld A, Sverdlik R C, Andrade L L(1974). Effects of hypothyroidism on serum immunoreactive insulin, free fatty acids and blood sugar in the dog as tested for oral glucose tolerance. Corrective effects of thyroxine therapy. Horm Metab Res 6:137.

Renauld A, Sverdlik R C, Andrade L L, Rodríguez R R(1975). Experimental hyperthyroidism in dogs. Evaluation and effects on blood sugar serum insulin and free fatty acids during glibenclamide infusion test. Horm Metab Res 7:382.

Shah J H, Cerchio G M(1973). Hypoinsulinemia of hypothyroidism. Arch Intern Med 132:657.

Sato K, Robbins J(1981). Thyroid hormone metabolism in primary cultured rat hepatocytes. Effects of glucose, glucagon and insulin. J Clin Invest 68:475.

Wallach S, Bellavia J, Gamponia P J, Bristrim P (1972). Thyroxine-induced simulation of hepatic cell transport of calcium and magnesium. J Clin Invest 51:1572.

Zamrazil V, Nedvidkova J, Felt V, Nemec J, Havelka J(1976). The influence of thyroid function on the diabetogenic action of triamcinolone in man. Glucose, insulin and growth hormone patterns after an oral glucose load. Horm Metab Res 8:282.

New Concepts in Thyroid Disease, pages 75–104

ADAPTATION TO IODINE DEFICIENCY IN THE LIGHT OF SOME NEWER CONCEPTS OF THYROID PHYSIOLOGY

J. Enrique Silva

Howard Hughes Medical Institute Laboratory and
Brigham and Women's Hospital, Dept. of Medicine
Harvard Medical School of Boston, Mass. U.S.A.

Iodine deficiency is still a major health problem in the world. Low iodine supply is a necessary condition - although not always the only one - for the development of endemic goiter. Among the many consequences that iodine deficiency and probably some accompanying conditions have on the people living in these areas, the most dreaded is endemic cretinism. Thus, while in non-deficient areas the incidence of congenital hypothyroidism is approximately 1 per 5000 births (Mitchel, M.L.,1978), in these endemic areas the prevalence of central nervous system damage presumably due to congenital and or intrauterine hypothyroidism may be as high as 15% (Phroah, P.,1980) and probably higher if less evident neurological sequelae were taken into consideration. On the other hand,the study of the impact of iodine deficiency on thyroid physiology as well as the response to this deficiency ,have provided for years an experimental and human model to understand the physiology of thyroid hormones. Likewise, iodine deficiency has stimulated the study of the effect of thyroid hormones on the development of the central nervous system.These specific studies as well as concepts developed recently have improved our understanding as to how the mammals cope with a low iodine intake as well as of the consequences that both the lack of iodine itself and the adaptation mechanisms to it have on human being.

The concepts developed in this Section are based on some widely accepted premises. One is that the effect of thyroid hormone is initiated in specific receptors located in the nucleus of the cells responsive to thyroid hormones (Oppenheimer, J.H.,1976). Since these receptors bind T_3 with much higher affinity (10-20 fold) than they do with T_4 and the latter is found in low concentration in the nuclei of target tissues (Surks,M.I., 1977), we assume that T_3 is ultimately the thyroid hormone. T_4 is basically a prohormone whose thyromimetic potency is accounted for almost completely by the T_3 that generates in various tissues. This concept, however, is valid only for physiological conditions since in situations where the concentration of T_4 is elevated to the point that occupies a significant fraction of the receptors, it may account for a significant fraction of the observed biological response, without being transformed in T_3. Other well accepted concept is that in normal conditions, at least 3/4 of the exchangeable extrathyroidal thyroidal T_3 is produced by 5'-deiodination of T_4 (McGuire, R.A., 1981). This figure is also valid for physiological conditions only since, as we will see later on, in various other situations, iodine deficiency among them, thyroid secretion may account for a greater fraction of the exchangeable T_3 pool.

In this section I will call adaptation to iodine deficiency to all those physiological and biochemical adjustments that ultimately result in the maintenance of the concentration of T_3 within the cells. These mechanisms are listed in Table 1. Both the increased capacity of the thyroid gland to clear iodine from plasma and the changes in the T_3/T_4 ratio in thyroid secretion have been known for years. The third mechanism has become evident from late studies of our group (Kaplan,M.M.,1980 - Leonard, J.L.,1981).

TABLE 1

Mechanism Ultimately Tending to keep Intracellular Concentration of Triiodothyronine in Iodine Deficiency

-- Increased thyroid clearance of plasma inorganic iodide

-- Enrichment of thyroid secretion in triiodothyronine

-- Enhanced thyroxine to triiodothyronine conversion in some tissues

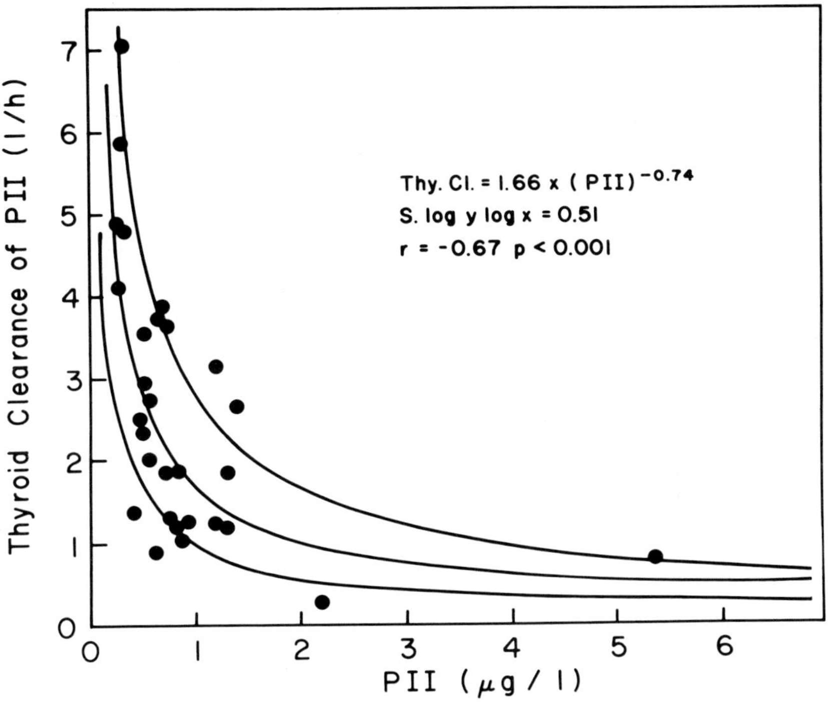

Fig. 1.- Relationship between thyroid clearance of plasma iodide and plasma iodide concentration. With data from Silva et al (1973). Rev Med Chile 101:763.

The clearance of plasma iodide by the gland as a function of the concentration of iodides in the serum is depicted in Fig. 1. These were studies performed in a moderately iodine deficient population in the central valley of Chile (Peumo) (Silva, J.E., 1973). These people had a mean urinary iodine excretion of approximately 35 ug/day. A clear inverse relationship between plasma inorganic iodide concentration (PII) and thyroid clearance (TC) was found. The relationship is such that the product of both, thyroid clearance and iodide concentration, elevated to an exponent of proportionality, is constant within the observed range of serum iodide concentration. This product represents the absolute iodine uptake (AIU), that is the mass of iodine available to the gland per unit of time. Since PII fluctuates very rapidly (Wayne, E.J., 1964), this finding indicates that adjustments of the clearance are also very rapid. The question is how the AIU compares with that from people without iodine deficiency, in other words, whether the mean increment ot TC showed by these iodine deficient people compensates for the mean observed fall in PII. Table II showes the AIU values obtained in this area according to the type of goiter.Figures from areas with higher iodine intake (Wayne, E.J., 1964 - De Groot, L.J., 1966) are given for comparison. The value of AIU tends to be lower in the iodine deficient area despite the elevated clearance indicating that this compensation may not be complete. Various studies (Oppenheimer, J.H.,1975 - Ibid, 1975 among others) allow to estimate the secretion of hormonal iodine in 60-70 ug/day in people with sufficient iodine intake. This figure is in agreement with the AIU of those two iodine sufficient populations given for comparison in Table 2 (Wayne, E.J., 1964 - De Groot, L.J., 1966). In contrast, the iodine deficient women had a value of only 45 ug/day which is even lower if those patients with multinodular goiter are excluded. The latter patients have indeed non-hormonal iodine "leak" from their goitrous glands (Barzelatto, J., 1967) which justifies their exclusion for comparison purposes. The low AIU value obtained in this iodine deficient population is in excellent agreement with the low production rate of T_4 found (39 $\pm$ ug/day) (Silva, J.E., 1971 - Stevenson, C., 1974) and the subsequent correction to 103 ug/day induced by iodine supplementation (Stevenson, C., 1974). Thus, whereas the thyroid gland can adjust the plasma clearance of iodide rapidly, the mean increase observed in TC does not fully compensate the mean fall in PII. The incapacity of fully compensating the low PII with an appropriate increase in TC probably accounts for the fall in iodine concentration in the glands of these subjects (Ermans, A.M., 1980) and in those of iodine deficient rats (Silva, J.E., 1972 - Abrams, G.M., 1973).

The effects of iodine deficiency in rats on thyroidal and on serum hormonal iodine are shown in Table 3 (Silva, J.E., 1972). It is well known that the distribution of the iodine in the thyroglobulin depends on the degree of iodination of the molecule. Low degrees of iodination decrease the proportion of DIT and as a consequence there is more MIT and T_3 relative to DIT and T_4. The thyroidal secretion is enriched in T_3. The latter is enhanced by TSH stimulation (Taurog, A., 1964) presumably by increase in

TABLE 2

Absolute Iodine Uptake in Subjects Living in an Iodine Deficient Area* (Mean $\pm$ SD)

	N	PII ug/1	T.C. 1/h	AIU ug/h
No Goiter	6	1.75 $\pm$ 0.6	1.75 $\pm$ 0.4	1.77 $\pm$ 0.4
Diffuse Goiter	13	0.69 $\pm$ 0.1	2.43 $\pm$ 0.4	1.63 $\pm$ 0.2
Nodular Goiter	10	0.74 $\pm$ 0.1	3.39 $\pm$ 0.6	2.30 $\pm$ 0.3
Reference data from non-goitrous areas				
De Groot ▲	4	3.50 $\pm$ 1.6	0.62 $\pm$ 0.2	2.20 $\pm$ 1.5
Wayne et al #	24	1.80 $\pm$ 0.1	1.24 $\pm$ 0.7	1.80 $\pm$ 0.8

* From Silva et al, 1973 . Rev. Med Chile 101:763. Daily urinary iodine excretion 36 $\pm$ 19 (SD) ug (Range 11.0 - 110 ug). All females, 56 $\pm$ 10 Kg (SD)

▲ From De Groot, 1966, J. Clin. Endocr. Metab. 26:149. Daily urinary iodide 128 $\pm$ 65 (SD). Three males, 1 female, 57-72 Kg.

From Wayne, Kontras Alexander, 1964. Clinical Aspects of Iodine Metabolism F.A. Davis Philadelphia. Daily urinary iodide 45 - 170 ug. All females, body weight not available.

T_4 to T_3 conversion occuring within the gland recently demostrated (Erickson, V.J., 1981). Thus 3 factors, an increase in the iodine turnover, a decrease in the degree of iodination of thyroglobulin and the effect of TSH, account for an augmented T_3 secretion. The studies shown in Table 3 were shortly corroborated by radioimmunoassay measurements of T_3 and T_4 concentration in the gland and in the serum of iodine deficient animals (Abrams, G.M., 1973). The serum concentration of T_3 was normal while that of T_4 was significantly decreased (Abrams, G.M., 1973). Since the

TABLE 3

Thyroidal and Serum Hormonal Iodine in Iodine Deficient Rats* (Mean ± SD; = 8-10/group)

Thyroid	Control	LID	P
Iodine Content # (ug/gland)	9.1 ± 0.8	1.0 ± 0.1	<0.001
Iodine Concentration (ug/mg wet tissue)	0.67 ± 0.05	0.03 ± 0.00	<0.001
T_4I (% total I) #	22.3 ± 1.0	18.2 ± 1.1	<0.002
T_4 (ug/gland)	3.4 ± 0.4	0.3 ± 0.0	<0.001
T_3I (% total I)	1.6 ± 0.1	8.0 ± 0.8	<0.001
T_3 (ug/gland)	0.23 ± 0.02	0.13 ± 0.02	<0.001
$T_3I/(T_4I + T_3I)$	6.7 ± 0.4	30.5 ± 2.5	<0.001
Serum			
Hormonal Iodine, H.I.▲ (ng/ml)	37.4 ± 1.6	13.6 ± 1.1	<0.001
$(T_4I/H.I)$ 100 #	97.5 ± 0.2	92.6 ± 1.1	<0.001
$(T_3/H.I.)$ 100 #	2.5 ± 0.2	7.4 ± 1.1	<0.001

LID = low iodine diet
* Data from Silva, J.E. (1972) Endocrinology 91:1430 and Silva , J.E. (1971) Mechanisms of adaptation to iodine deficiency in man and rat. University of Chile. Postgraduate Thesis
# Rats were isotopically equilibrated as described by Silva, J.E. (1972) Endocrinology 91:1430. Thyroid digestion and iodoaminoacids chromatography were performed as described by Inoue and Taurog (1967) Endocrinology 81:319. The mass of hormones was calculated from specific activity of the diet. The latter was equal to that of thyroidal iodine indicating

complete equilibration.
▲ Hormonal iodine was determined by cation exchange chromatography as per Backer et al (1967) Clin. Chim. Acta 15:77.

metabolic clearance rate of both hormones was not altered by the iodine deficiency (Silva, J.E., 1972), the production rate was well reflected by their serum concentration. Because of the lack of change in the fractional turnover of T_4 (Silva, J.E., 1972), the overall fractional T_4 to T_3 conversion rate is expected to be unaltered, as it has been found to be the case in liver and kidney from iodine deficient rats (unpublished observation). Therefore, the normal level of T_3 has to be explained on the basis of increased thyroidal secretion (Abrams,G.M., 1973 - Silva,J.E., 1974). Similar findings have been obtained in humans living in endemic goiter areas (Silva, J.E.,1974 - Ermans, A.M., 1968).

Under normal circumstances about 35-40 % of the T_4 is converted to T_3, 40 % is degraded to the inactive metabolite 3',5',3triiodothyronine (reverse T_3, rT_3) and the remainder 20% is excreted in the feces conjugated mainly to glucoronic acid (Ibid 1975). Thus, if normally 3/4 of T_3 come from peripheral 5'- deiodination of about 40% of the T_4 daily production rate, in order to produce approximately 24 ug of T_3, equivalent to 14 ug of iodine (approximately 3/4 of the total daily production rate), the thyroid gland should secrete 80 ug of T_4 or 52 ug of iodine. Therefore, the shift of T_3 source from peripheral production to thyroidal secretion decreases the functional burden of the gland to keep the AIU normal. If all daily production of T_3 was secreted, the AIU could decrease about 38 ug daily, (=52 ug IT_4 - 14 ug I T_3 produced peripherally from T_4 5'-deiodination and now secreted by the gland).The observed fall in AIU in iodine deficient population may thus be accounted for by this shift of the T_3 production from peripheral towards thyroidal.

How are these changes possible ? What consequences do they have for tissue supply of T_3 ? The discovery of T_3 nuclear receptors, the relative affinity for T_3, the relatively small amount of T_4 found in the nucleus and the observation that the metabolic effect of T_4 can be blunted by blocking its conversion to T_3, are the fundamentals to think that ultimately T_3 is the thyroid hormone (Table 4). This view is in good agreement with the clinical impression that subjects

TABLE 4

Evidence that Triiodothyronine Accounts for Most if Not All The Biological Activity of Thyroid Secretion

-- Biological potency and time course of the effect as compared to that of thyroxine

-- Affinity of nuclear receptors is at least 10 times greater for triiodothyronine than for thyroxine

-- The amount of thyroxine specifically bound to these receptors is 10% or less of the nuclear iodothyronines

-- The blockade of thyroxine to triiodothyronine conversion decreases markedly the biological effect of thyroxine

with endemic goiter are clinically euthyroid since serum T_3 is normal or even slightly elevated (Goslings, B.M., 1977 - Chopra, I.J., 1977) in them. To address this question I studied some biological responses to thyroid hormones in chronically iodine deficient rats. As shown in Table 3, these rats had greater than 90% depletion of thyroidal iodine but they had normal T_3 production rate and subnormal T_4 secretion (Fig. 2) (Silva, J.E., 1972). Fig. 3 and 4 show that none of the variables studied, growth rate, basal oxygen consumption, metabolic response to cold, were affected by this fall in thyroxine production (Silva, J.E., 1972). More recently, it has been shown that hepatic alfa-glycero-phosphate dehydrogesase activity, a thyroid hormone responsive enzyme may be decreased, but in animals with a substantially more severe iodine depletion (Okamura, K., 1981 - Riesco, G., 1977), in one study as severe as to decrease serum T_3 (Riesco, G., 1977). However, the studies illustrated in Figs 2, 3 and 4 and in Table 3, are probably more comparable to the degree of deficiency observed in the human. At any rate, these studies are in agreement with the view that T_3 accounts for most of the biological potency of thyroid secretion. Yet, there was an apparently major discrepancy with this view. In iodine deficiency as well as in other conditions such as early stages of Hashimoto's thyroiditis, hypothyroidism post

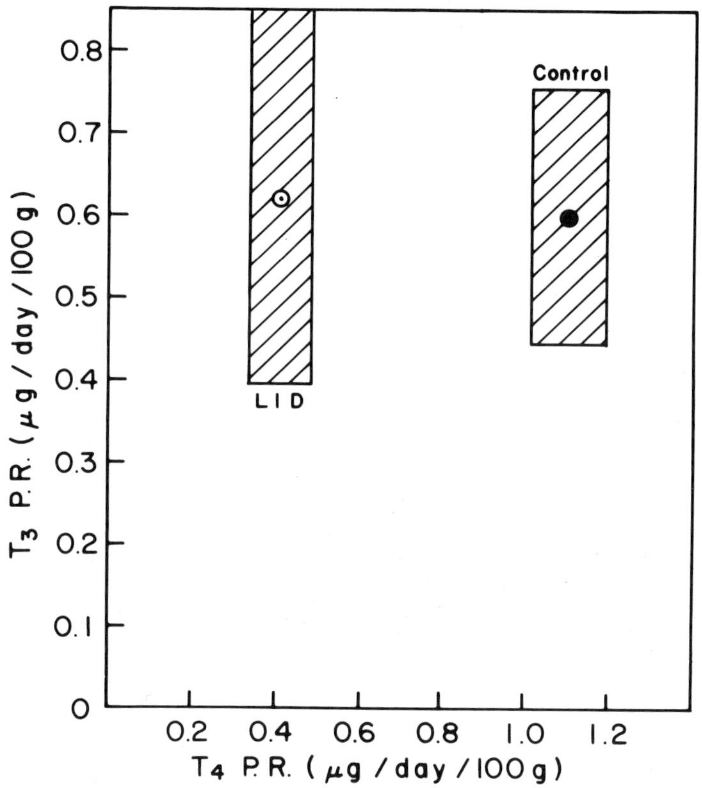

Fig. 2.- Production rates of T_4 and T_3 in iodine deficient rats (LID). Data from J. E. Silva (1972) Endocrinology 91:1430, and J. E. Silva (1971) Mechanisms of adaptation to iodine deficiency in man and rat. University of Chile Postgraduate Thesis.

radioactive iodine or surgery, subjects with normal serum T_3 and low T_4, have levels of serum TSH general markedly elevated, although they are clinically euthyroid and, as shown above, it is difficult to demonstrate biochemical evidence of hypothyroidism. This elevation of TSH has also been found in experimental animals (Fukuda, H., 1975 - Riesco, G., 1977). Serum TSH seems to correlate much better with serum T_4 (Chopra, I.J., 1977) so that, when the latter is low, the pituitary seem to be hypothyroid while all or

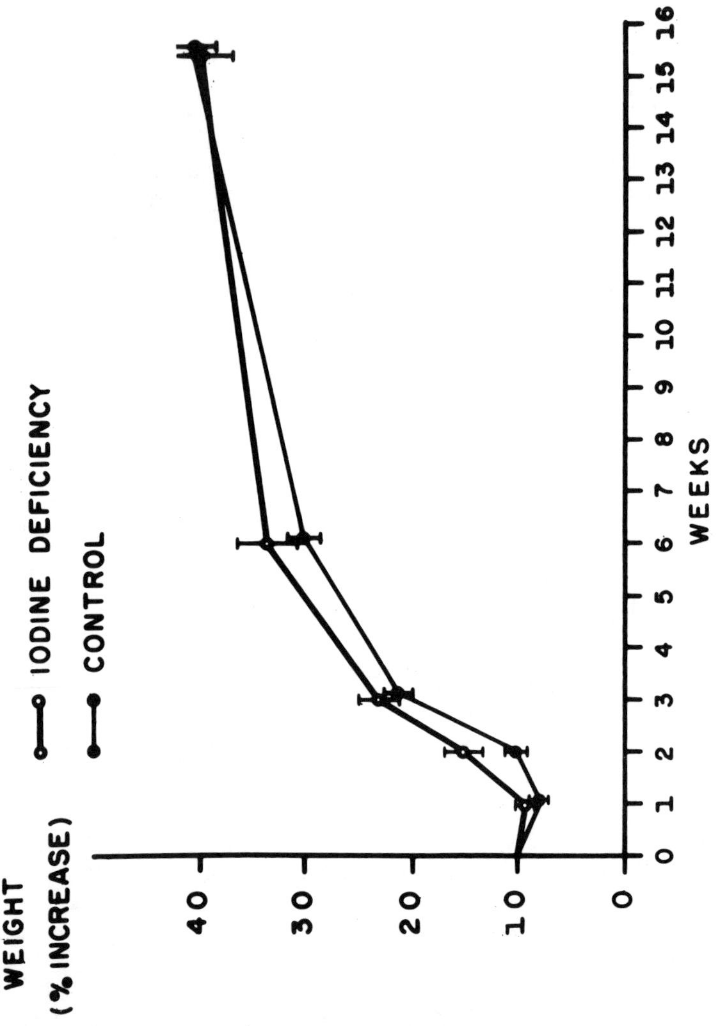

Fig. 3.- Weight increase of iodine deficient rats. Both groups received the same diet. Control group's diet was supplemented with KI to 0.79 ug/g. Each value is the mean + SEM of ten rats. (From J.E. Silva (1972) Endocrinology 91:1430 - with permission of the editor)

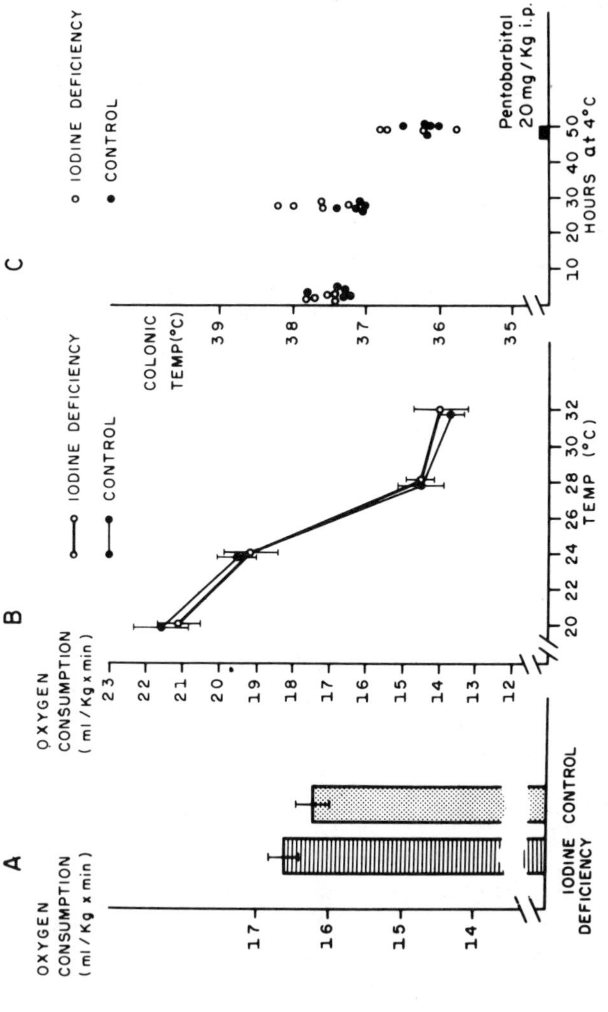

Fig. 4.- A.Oxygen consumption at 28 C. Values are the mean + SE of 20 measurements in each group of 5 rats. B. Oxygen consumption at different environmental temperatures. Values are the mean + SE of 16 (iodine deficiency) or 20 (controls) measurements in groups of 5 rats each. C. Colonic temperatures of rats at 4 + 2 C environmental temperature. Each point represents one rat. The last values were obtained after 2 hr of anesthesia

with pentobarbital. Iodine deficient rats received Remington diet with 0.093 ug/^{127}I/g during three months. The control group was on the same diet supplemented with KI (final ^{127}I concentration:0.793 ug/g)., (From J.E. Silva (1972) Endocrinology 91:1430, with permission of the Editor).

most other tissues do not seem to be significantly hypothyroid, provided serum T_3 is within normal limits.

A few years ago we showed that the effect of T_4 on TSH release inhibition is only apparent (Silva, J.E., 1977). TSH inhibition, as most of biological responses to T_3, seems to be a nuclear mediated effect and therefore, it is possible to correlate T_3 - induced TSH suppression with the nuclear T_3 content in anterior pituitary cells (Silva, J.E., 1978). We demonstrated that besides the chronological relation between nuclear events and TSH suppression (Silva,J.E., 1977), there is a linear relationship between nuclear occupancy by T_3 and TSH suppression as shown in Fig. 5 (Silva, J.E., 1978). Furthermore, we demonstrated that T_4-induced TSH suppression correlated with the amount of T_3 generated locally from T_4 and subsequently bound to the nucleus (Silva, J.E., 1977 - Silva, J.E., 1978). There was no T_4 specifically bound to nuclear receptors (Silva, J.E., 1978) nor did we find specific high affinity receptors for T_4 somewhere else in the tissue. Most importantly, the bulk T_3 generated from T_3 and found specifically bound to nuclear receptors, was generated inside of the cell. Only a minor portion was produced in other tissues and entered the adenohypophysis via plasma (Silva, J.E., 1977 -Silva, J.E., 1978). The relevance of the intracellularly generated T_3 from T_4, T_3 (T_4), in suppressing TSH was further demonstrated by the blockade of T_4 effect with Iopanoic acid, a constrast medium used for cholecystography (Larsen, P.R., 1979). This iodinated compound blocks competitively the enzymatically mediated T_4 to T_3 conversion (Kaplan, M.M., 1978). In these experiments while iopanoic acid did not block the suppresive effect of T_3 on TSH release, it did abolish that of T_4, although the concentration of T_4 in the serum did not fall (Larsen, P.R., 1979). Studying euthyroid rats with isotopic dilution techniques explained in another section of this book, we were able to determine that while in liver and kidney, two typical thyroid hormone responsive tissues, most of nuclear T_3 came from plasma T_3, in the pituitary a half of the nuclear T_3 came from this source while the other half was locally generated from T_4

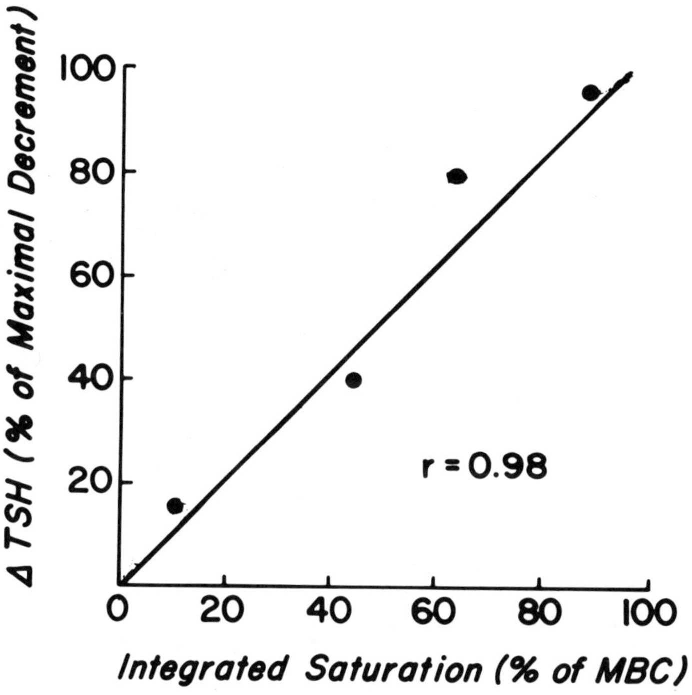

Fig. 5.-Relationship between nuclear occupancy by T_3 in the anterior pituitary and TSH suppression. Thyroidectomized rats were injected with increasing doses of T_3 and killed 3 hours later. The integrated nuclear ocupancy was calculated from the time course of nuclear T_3 binding (in a parallel experiment), the plasma and nuclear radioactive T_3 and the specific activity of the injected doses.

(Silva, J.E., 1978) as shown in Table 5. These findings provided an excellent explanation for the observations alluded to in iodine deficiency in the paragraph above, namely, lack of evidence of hypothyroidism, normal T_3, low T_4 and elevated TSH. Thus, while a fall in serum T_4 would not give rise to a major, detectable, desaturation of nuclear sites in liver, heart, skeletal muscle, all thyroid hormone responsive tissues and responsible for most of the clinical manifestations of thyroid disfunction, it would produce a

TABLE 5

Estimated Contributions of Plasma Triiodothyronine (T3) and Intracellular Thyroxine (T4) Deiodination to T3 to Nuclear T3 of Anterior Pituitary, Liver and Kidney of Euthyroid Rats

NT_3 (ng T_3/mg DNA)[a]	Anterior Pituitary	Liver	Kidney
From plasma T_3, T_3 (T3)	0.29	0.13	0.06
From local T_4 monodeiodination, T_3 (T_4)	0.31	0.05	0.01
Total NT_3	0.60	0.18	0.07
MBC	0.77	0.37	0.13
% Saturation	78	48	53

[a]Based on mean ($\pm$ SD) plasma T_4 of 2.9 $\pm$ 0.8 ug/dl and T_3 of 48 $\pm$ ng/dl in these rats. The concentration of NT_3 was calculated multiplying these values by the NT_3 (T3): plasma T_3 (^{131}I-T3) and NT_3 (T4): plasma T_4 (^{125}I T3/^{125}I T4) ratios obtained at equilibrium after the injection of the tracers.
MBC = Maximal binding capacity of T3 in ng/mg DNA
Data from Silva et al (1978) Endocrinology 103:1196

significant depletion of nuclear T_3 in the pituitary. The fall in serum T_4, reflection of thyroidal iodine depletion, will cause a fall in peripheral T_3 production. However, the increase in serum TSH along with the changes described in thyroidal iodine will compensate for this fall in peripheral production of T_3 with a proportional increase in thyroidal T_3 secretion. These adjustments occurring in iodine deficiency as well as in other conditions of failing thyroid gland are illustrated in Fig. 6.

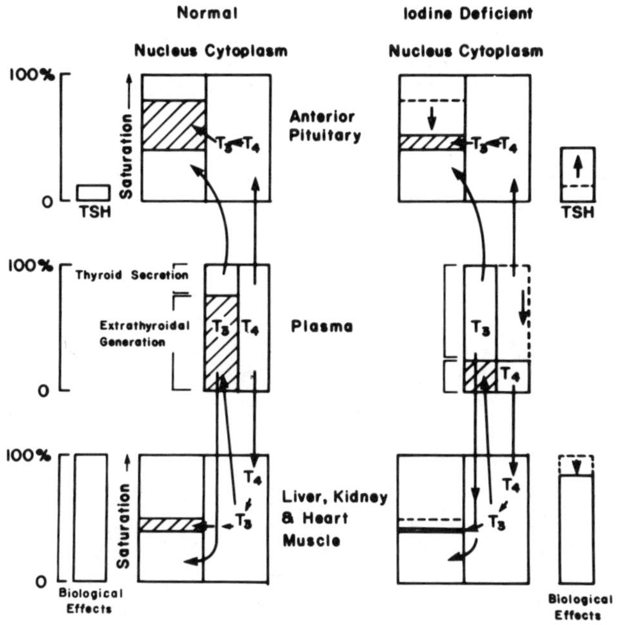

Fig. 6.-Adapted from J.E. Silva (1979) Rev Med Chile 107:950. On the left side is diagramatically represented the normal situation. The nuclear receptors in the pituitary are 80-90% saturated and half of this nuclear T3 is produced locally from T4 deiodination; the remainder is borne via plasma. Other major target tissues of thyroid hormone are approximately 50% saturated and 25% or less of this T3 is produced locally; the remainder, although it may be produced at a great extent in these tissues, exchanges actively with plasma so that the amount of T3 derived from this source is a direct function of plasma T3

concentration.The diagram of plasma T3 and T4 illustrates that 3/4 of serum T3 are normally produced from T4 outside of the thyroid. In iodine deficiency and other conditions of diminished thyroid reserve, the fall in serum thyroid hormones drives the pituitary. As a consequence of TSH stimulation and low thyroidal iodine concentration, the thyroid secretion is enriched in T3. As a result of these changes the bulk of plasma T3 is now secreted and the serum level of T3 is normal. Liver, kidney, heart, skeletal muscle and other tissues have almost a normal supply of T3 and therefore they are euthyroid or minimally hypothyroid.On the other hand, the pituitary is significantly depleted of T3 because of the shortage of T4. This tissue is hypothyroid but this mechanism protects other more vital organs from the lack of thyroid hormone.

The adaptation described seems to be quite efficient. There are however circumstances where these mechanisms may not operate as efficiently. For example, Table 6, taken from Dussault and Walker (1978), shows that newborn rats whose mothers have been subjected to an iodine deficient diet during pregnancy, are born with undetectable T_4 and T_3 whereas, as it has been shown above, the adult iodine deficient rat keeps normal the serum concentration of T_3. This indicates that an immature pituitary thyroid system, as it is that of the rat compared to the human one at birth, may not be able to adapt efficiently to iodine deficiency. Stages comparable to these may occur in the human in utero and may account, at least in part, for the high frequency of central nervous system damage observed in areas of endemic goiter (Mitchel,M.L., 1978 - Phroah, P., 1980). Likewise, women well adapted to iodine deficiency when they become pregnant may decompensate. Table 7 summarizes the factors of higher iodine requirement during pregnancy and lactation. Normally,the thyroid gland competes with kidney for PII. Renal clearance is relatively fixed, independent of PII and similar in magnitude to the thyroid clearance when the iodine intake is within safe limits (Silva, J.E., 1973 - Wayne, E.J. 1964). Because of poorly understood reasons but probably through estrogen mediated mechanisms, the renal clearance of iodine increases significantly during pregnancy (Hollingsworth D., 1980) and hence the urinary losses of iodine. On the other hand, the fetal thyroidal iodine pool starts to be formed around the third month of gestation. If at birth the newborn iodine pool is 3.5mg and the mother iodine intake

TABLE 6

How Efficient is Adaptation to iodine deficiency
During Gestation?

New Born Iodine Deficient Rats

	T_4 ug/dl	T_3 ng/dl	TSH ng/ml
Birth			
LID	N.D.	N.D.	1140 ± 210
Control	0.5 ± 0.01	4.1 ± 0.2	221 ± 22
Age 18 Days			
LID	2.9 ± 0.3	110 ± 2.1	2160 ± 320
Control	5.9 ± 0.6	44 ± 3.2	390 ± 40

Mean ± SEM
LID = low iodine diet
N.D. = non-detectable
From Dussault and Walker (1978) Canadian J. Physiol. 56:950

has been 35 ug/day throughout pregnancy, the burden of forming the fetal pool is equal to 100 days with no iodine intake for the mother. A significant further fall in PII is expected in iodine deficient pregnant women that may well not be compensated by a further proportional increase in thyroidal plasma clearance of inorganic iodine.

Table 8 shows the serum levels of total T_4, T_3 and TSH in pregnant women and in cord blood of newborn from a moderately deficient area of South East Greater Santiago. The frequency distribution of urinary iodide is shown in Fig. 7. The observations were made between 10 weeks gestation through delivery. Gestational age during this period did not influence any of the hormone level measured (Silva, J.E., 1981) probably because at approximately 10-12 weeks the level of Thyroxine Binding Globulin (TBG) reaches a plateau (Fisher,

TABLE 7

Factors that increase daily iodine requirements during Gestation and Lactation

-- Formation of fetal iodine pool

-- Increased renal clearance of plasma iodide

-- Expanded thyroxine and triiodothyronine pools (Increase in plasma binding; only transient increased demand during first trimester).

-- Iodine excretion in the milk

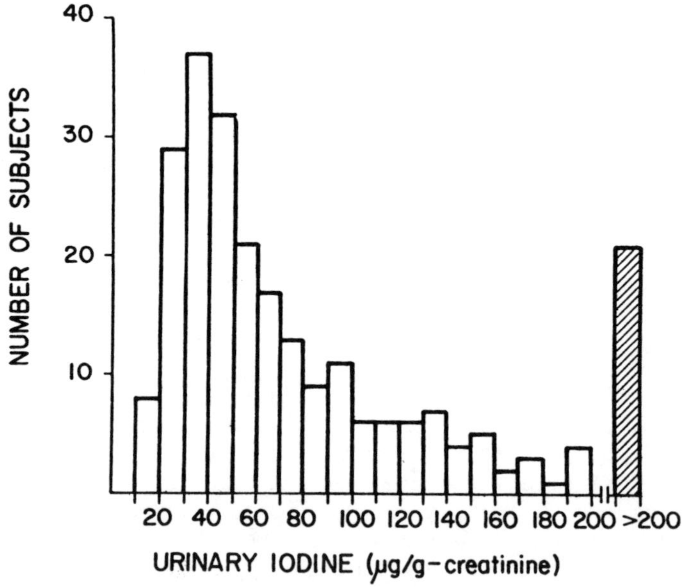

Fig. 7.- Urinary iodine excretion in 250 pregnant women in an iodine deficient area. ▨ About 8% of the subjects who had a urinary iodine level greater than 200 ug/g cr. (From Silva (1981) J. Clin. Endocrin. 52:671, with permission of the Editor).

TABLE 8

Serum Thyroid Hormone Levels in 12 - 40 Week Pregnant Women and in Cord Blood of Newborns in an area of moderate iodine deficiency (mean $\pm$ SD)

	T_4 ug/dl	T_3 ng/dl	rT_3 ng/dl	TSH uU/ml
A - Pregnant Women	8.9 ± 0.7	179 ± 45	25 ± 9	2.9 ± 1.7
	(247)	(245)	(95)	(249)
B - Newborn	8.6 ± 2.1	41 ± 23	172 ± 63	8.3 ± 6.0
	(208)	(211)	(119)	(208)

Urinary iodine excretion of these women is presented in Fig. 7. Urinary iodide of the mothers whose newborn were sampled were not always available. The few paired studies that were possible are presented in Table 11. Newborns are normal with estimated age at birth of 40 ± 2 weeks and weighing $>$2800g. The numbers in parenthesis indicate the number of samples tested.

D.A., 1974). As evident in Table 8, the expected increase in total serum T_4 was not observed since the value obtained is lower than those reported in areas with normal iodine intake ranging 9 - 15 ug/dl (Abuid, J.,1976 - Burrow, G.N., 1975). However, serum T_3 did increase in proportion to the elevation in plasma binding. In order to test this hypothesis and rule out other factors that could explain the failure of serum T_4 to augment in proportion TGB, these women were given 300 ug I/day as KI drops and they were observed a minimum of 4 weeks later (Silva, J.E., 1981). The results are shown in Tables 9 and 10. The dialyzable fraction of T_4 and T_3 underwent the expected fall due to the increase in TGB. Since total T_4 did not increase, a low free T_4 concentration was observed but the free serum T_3 concentration was normal because the level of total serum T_3 increased in proportion to the level of TGB. With the supplement of iodine given, a significant increase in both total and free serum T_4 was observed,indicating that the lack of iodine was responsible for the failure of T_4 to increase. Most interestingly, total and free serum T_3 did not change and TSH fell slightly but significantly ($p < 0.001$). Reverse T_3 also increased modestly but significantly. These observations are in excellent agreement with the discussion above and with the model illustrated in Fig. 5. Thus, before iodine supplementation the level of serum free T_4 was low and this elicited an increase in TSH. The diminished T_3 formation resulting from the decreased availability of substrate, (T_4), was compensated by an increase in thyroidal T_3 secretion. When iodine was given, extrathyroidal T_3 production normalized because the concentration of T_4 attained a normal value. TSH production also returned to normal and so did the thyroidal secretion of T_3. This in turn indicates that with a normal thyroid gland, the small change observed in serum TSH (1.8 uU/ml in average) is physiologically relevant (Silva, J.E., 1981).

Table 11 shows the effects of iodine deficiency in the cord blood level of thyroid hormones. For obvious reasons, this was an unpaired study at variance with that described in the paragraph above. The newborn of mothers with moderate iodine deficiency had low levels of T_4 when compared with newborns from areas of normal iodine supply (Abuid, J., 1976). This view is supported by the fact that a physiological supply of iodine given to the mothers resulted in values of cord serum T_4 comparable to those found in non-deficient areas. Serum T_3 in the newborn was not affected by maternal iodine intake. The relevance of these observations is still unclear.

TABLE 9

Effect of Iodine Supplementation on Serum Thyroid Hormones and TSH Concentrations during Pregnancy (Mean ± SD)

	urinary iodide	T_4	T_3	RT_3	TSH	Range GA*	Observation time interval
	ug/g-cr*	ug/dl	ng/dl	ng/dl	uU/ml	weeks	weeks
TREATED MOTHERS (N=36)							
Basal	53±33	8.7±2.4	187±25	21±7	2.8±1.4	9-32	
KI*	376±456	12.5±1.8	180±46	25±9	1.5±0.8	15-40	4-16
Change	+323±450	+3.8±2.2	-7±46	+4±10	-1.3±1.5		
p‡	<0.001	<0.001	N.S.	<0.02	<0.001		
UNTREATED CONTROLS (N=10)							
Basal	54±36	9.4±2.2	179±33	22±7	3.0±2.1	11-30	
End Observation	56±25	9.3±2.6	165±36	24±8	2.6±1.6	21-40	4-16
Change	-2±18	-0.1±2.8	-14±43	+2±9	-0.4±0.25		
p	N.S.	N.S.	N.S.	N.S.	N.S.		

* ug of iodine per gram of urinary creatinine
* G.A. = gestational age
* KI = Potassium iodide ≃300 ug I/day p.o.
‡ = paired t test

Data from Silva and Silva (1981) J. Clin. Endocrin. Metab. 52:671

TABLE 10

Serum free T4 and T3 concentration in iodine-deficient pregnant women:effect of iodine supplementation (mean+SD)

	T4 (ng/dl)	Free fraction (%x10^{3})	Free T4 (ng/dl)	T3 (ng/dl)	Free fraction (%x10^{2})	Free T3 (ng/dl)	TSH (uU/ml)
1.Nonpregnant adult (n=14)	7.7±1.8	30±5	2.3±0.4	124±26	28±4	0.34±0.14	5
2.Pregnant before OIS (n=14)	8.1±2.5	20±4[a]	1.5±0.4[a]	184±25[a]	18±4[a]	0.33±0.06	3.0±1.3
3.Pregnant after OIS (n=14)	12.2±1.9[a]	19±3[a]	2.3±0.4	177±38[b]	17±2[a]	0.30±0.06	1.2±0.6
P 2 vs 3 (paired)	<0.001	NS	<0.001	NS	NS	NS	<0.001

[a] $p < 0.001$ vs. nonpregnant control.

[b] $p <$ p.005 vs. nonpregnant control.

OIS = oral iodine supplementation as described in Table 9

Data from Silva and Silva (1981) J. Clin. Endocrinol. Metab 52:671

TABLE 11

Effect of Maternal Iodine Supplementation on Thyroid Hormones and TSH Concentrations in cord sera (Mean + SD)

	T_4 ug/dl	$D.F.T_4$ % X 10^{-2}	FT_4 ng/dl	T_3 ng/dl	$D.F.T_3$ % X 10^{-2}	FT_3 ng/dl	RT_3 ng/dl	TSH uU/ml
Untreated	9.3±1.7	2.4±0.3	2.2±0.4	50±23	24±3	0.13±0.05	183±37	8.3±7.8
	(32)	(16)	(16)	(33)	(17)	(17)	(34)	(34)
Treated	11.3±1.5	2.5±06	2.9±0.7	58±8	25±3	0.12±0.4	226±55	5.7±3.4
	(24)	(19)	(19)	(23)	(19)	(19)	(25)	(25)
% change	+22	+4	+32	+16	+4	-8	+24	-31
	<0.001	NS	<0.001	NS	NS	NS	<0.005	NS

DFT_4 or DFT_3 = Dialysable fraction

FT_4 or FT_3 = Free Hormone concentration

RT_3 = Total serum Reverse $-T_3$ concentration

Number of cases in parenthesis

Data from Silva and Silva (1981) J. Clin. Endocrinol. Metab. 52:671

On the one hand, this means that a kind of adaptation is observed in the newborn similar to that observed in the adult, and one might conclude that the human fetus is able to compensate adequately a moderately low iodine intake. On the other hand, we have recently demonstrated that in the cerebral cortex of the rat, about 80% of the nuclear T_3 is derived from cortical T_4 to T_3 conversion whereas only 20% is provided by plasma T_3 (Crantz, F.R., 1980 - Crantz, F.R., 1981).On this basis, one could think that the observed fall in cord serum T_4 is not trivial since it may result in a significant fall in cerebral T_3. Furthermore, we do not know if the compensation has been achieved only shortly before birth and one could think that in early stages during fetal life, both T_3 and T_4 are decreased, as suggested by the findings in newborn iodine deficient rats (Table 5, Hollingsworth, D., 1980). The short supply of thyroid hormone during this period, in this case most importantly of T_4, may thus have consequences for brain development. The situation, however, seems to be more complex. Dr Kaplan in our laboratory has found that the 5'- deiodinase activity in vitro is increased in hypothyroidism (Kaplan, M.M., 1980 - Kaplan, M.M., 1980), suggesting that a compensatory increase in T_4 to T_3 conversion could take place in conditions like this. Moreover, the brain seems to respond very rapidly in this respect to a fall in thyroid hormone concentration in the serum (Leonard, J.L., 1981). In order to test the hypothesis whether a decrease in the level of T_4 and/or T_3 could induce changes in the activity of this enzyme in some tissues, particularly the brain, we have performed experiments in newborn rats with various degrees of hypothyroidism induced by graded doses of methylmercaptoimidazol (MMI) in the drinking water of pregnant and subsequently nursing rats. As shown in Fig.8, rats whose mothers received the intermediate concentration of MMI have normal serum T_3 but decreased T_4, as observed in iodine deficiency. In these rats a striking increase in T_4 to T_3 conversion was observed in the cerebral cortex while the liver showed a change in the opposite direction. These preliminary studies, as we have recently suggested, (Larsen. P.R., 1981) are further evidence that there may be mechanisms at cellular level that regulate the intracellular concentration of T_3. These mechanisms are operative in conditions such as iodine deficiency when the T_4 concentration in the serum is decreased and, most interestingly, they seem to take place in tissues that depend more heavily - such as the brain - on T_4 supply for their intracellular content of T_3.

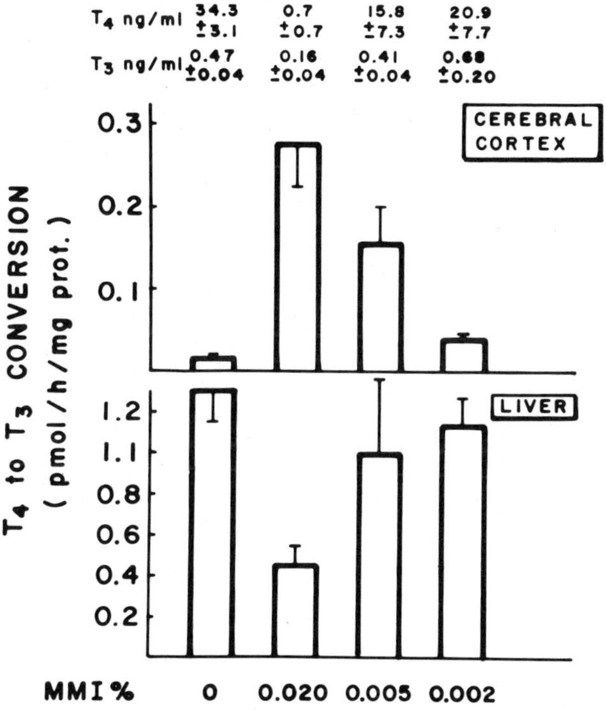

Fig. 8.-Pregnant rats were given MMI in indicated concentrations from day 16th of gestational age throughout lactation. Groups of 4-5 pups were killed at 2 weeks. T4 to T3 conversion was assayed in vitro in crude homogenates, with 2 mM ^{125}I T4 and 20 mM Dithiothreitol DTT (cortex) or 1 mM DTT (Liver). T4 and T3 serum concentrations (RIA) for each group are shown on the top of the figure.

In brief, adaptation to iodine deficiency defined as the mechanisms resulting in the maintenance of normal intracellular levels of T_3, takes place at several levels. The capacity of the thyroid gland to concentrate iodine is increased but the larger volume of plasma cleared of iodide does not seem to fully compensate for the fall in PII. The ensuing reduction in the degrees of iodination of thyroglobulin results in decreased content of T_4 and hence decreased serum T_4. Because of the important contribution of intrapituitary T_4 to T_3 conversion to intracellular T_3 in the pituitary, this gland undergoes a significant depletion of T_3 that gives rise to an increase in TSH secretion. Both, the low level of iodination of thyroglobulin and TSH stimulation of the thyroid result in augmented thyroidal secretion of T_3 that compensates for the decrease in extra-thyroidal production derived from the reduced pool of T_4. The serum T_3 concentration is thus maintained within normal limits. Since most tissues responsive to thyroid hormone depend on serum T_3 for their T_3 supply, few or none metabolic manifestations of hypothyroidism can be demonstrated. Lastly, tissues highly dependent on T_4 for their intracellular content of T_3 like the brain, undergo a significant increase in T_4 to T_3 conversion. The regulation of TSH secretion under these circumstances and the changes in tissue generation of T_3 from 5'-deiodination of T_4 are mechanisms probably operative in other circumstances of reduced thyroidal functional reserve as well.

ACKNOWLEDGEMENTS

Most of the studies shown have been done in Chile with support of CONICYT Grant #165, 1969 and from the Comision de Investigación Científica de la U de Chile M 144792. The author is indebted to all whose dedicated technical assistance made this work possible, Mrs. C. Jara, C. Keitel, M. Larrondo L. Madariaga, E. Madrid, and Mr. Hernan Riquelme. The studies on TSH regulation and on sources of cellular T_3 have been done in Howard Hughes Medical Institute Laboratory in Boston USA under the direction of Dr P. Reed Larsen to whom I am also deeply indebted. The careful secretarial work of Ms. Faith Baldwin is also well appreciated, as well as the technical assistance of T.E. Dick, S. Mellen and G. Weiss in Boston, Mass. USA.

REFERENCES

Abrams, G.M., Larsen, P.R. (1973) Triiodothyronine and thyroxine in the serum and thyroid glands of iodine deficient rats. J. Clin. Invest 52:2522

Abuid, J., Klein, A.H., Foley, T.P., Jr., and Larsen, P.R. (1976) Total and free triiodothyronine and thyroxine in early infancy. J. Clin. Endocrin 39:263

Barzelatto, J., Beckers, C., Stevenson, C., Covarrubias, E., Gianetti, A, Bobdilla, E., Pardo, A., Donoso, H., and Atria, A. (1967) Endemic goiter in Pedregoso (Chile) I. description and function studies. Acta Endocrinológica (Kbh) 54:577.

Burrow, G.N., Polackwich, R. and Domabedian, R. (1975) The hypothalamic pituitary axis in normal pregnancy in: Preinatal Thyroid Physiology and Disease D.A.Fisher and G.N.Burrows (Eds) Raven Press, New York, page 1.

Crantz, F.R., Larsen, P.R. (1980) Rapid thyroxine to 3,5,3' triiodothyronine conversation and nuclear 3,5,3'-triiodothyronine binding in rat cerebral cortex and cerebellum J. Clin. Invest 65:935

Crantz,F.R., Silva, J.E., and Larsen, P.R. (1981) An analysis of the sources and quantity of 3,5,3'- triiodothyronine specifically bound to nuclear receptors in rat cerebral cortex and cerebellum. Endocrinology, In press.

Chopra, I.J., D.H., Solomon and G.N. Chua Teco. Thyroxine: Just a prohormone too? J. Clin, Endocrinol Metab. 44:481, 1977

De Groot, L.J. (1966) Kinetic analysis of iodine metabolism. J. Clin. Endocrinol. Metab 26:149

Dussault, J.H.,and Walker, P., (1978) Hypothalamic TRH concentrations in neonatal rats exposed to PTU and low iodine diet. Canadian J. Physiol 56:950

Ermans, A.M. (1980) Ethiopathogenesis of endemic goiter. In: Endemic Goiter and Cretinism J.B.Stanbury and B.S.Hetzel (Eds) John Wiley and Sons Inc. New York page 287

Ermans, A.M.,Kinthaert, J., Delcroix, C., and Collard, J. (1968). Metabolism of intrathyroidal iodine in normal men. J. Clin. Endocrinol. 28:169, 1968

Erickson, V.J., Calcieri, R.R., and Rosenberg, L.L. (1981) Phenolic and non-phenolic ring iodothyronine deiodinases from rat thyroid gland. Endocrinology 108:1257

Fisher, D.A., and Dussault, J.H. (1974) Development of the mammilian thyroid gland. In: Handbook of Physiology Section 7 Endocrinology Volume III: Thyroid American Physiol Society Washington, D.C. R.O. Greep and E.B. Ostwood Eds.

page 21.
Fukuda, H., Yasuda, N., Greer, M.A., Kutas, M., Greer, S.E. (1975) Changes in plasma thyroxine, triiodothyronine, and TSH during adaptation to iodine deficiency in the rat. Endocrinology 97:307
Goslings, B.M., Djokomowljanto, R., Docter, C., van Hardeveld, G., Hennemann,D., Smeenk, and A. Querido. Hypothyroidism in an area of endemic goiter and cretinism in central Java, Indonesia J. Clin. Endocrinol Metab. 44:481, 1977
Hollingsworth, D., Fisher, D.A., Pretell, E.A. (1980) The fetal maternal relationship with respect to the thyroid. In: Stanbury, J.B., Hetzel, B.S. (eds) Endemic Goiter and Endemic Cretinism. John Wiley and Sons, New York, page 423.
Ibid (1975) Erratum: Revised calculations of common parameters of iodothyronine metabolism and distribution in man by noncompartmental analysis. J. Clin. Endocrinol Metab. 41:1175
Kaplan, M.M.,(1980) Thyroxine 5'-monodeiodination in rat anterior pituitary homogenates. Endocrinology 106:567
Kaplan, M.M. and Yaskoski, K.A. (1980) Phenolic and tyrosyl ring iodothyronine deiodination in rat brain nomogenates J. Clin. Invest. 66:551
Kaplan, M.M.,Utiger, R.D. (1978) Iodothyronine metabolism in rat liver homogenates. J. Clin Invest 61:459
Leonard, J.L., Kaplan, M.M., Visser, T.J., Silva, J.E., and Larsen, P.R. (1981) Cerebral Cortex responds rapidly to thyroid hormones Science 214:571
Larsen, PR, Dick,T.E., Markovitz, B.P., Kaplan, M.M., Gard, T.G. (1979) Inhibition of intrapituitary thyroxine to 3,5,3' triiodothyronine conversion prevents the acute suppression of thyrotropin release by thyroxine in hypothyroid rats. J.Clin Invest 64:117
Larsen, P.R., Silva, J.E., and Kaplan, M.M. (1981) Relationships between circulating and intracellular thyroid hormones: physiological and clinical implications Endocrine Reviews 2:87
Mitchel, M.L.,Larsen, P.R., Levy, H.L., Bennett, A.J.E. and Madoff, M.A.(1978) Screening for congenital hypothyroidism J. American Med Assn. 239:2348
McGuire,R.A., and Hays, M.T. (1981) A kinetic model of human thyroid hormones and their conversion products J Clin Endocrinol Metab 53:852
Oppenheimer,J.H., Schwartz, H.L., Surks, M.I., Koerner, D., Dillmann, W.H.(1976) Nuclear receptors and the initiation of thyroid hormone action. Recent Prog Horm Res 32:529
Oppenheimer, J.H,,Schwartz, H.L., and Surks, M.I. (1975)

Determination of Common Parameters of Iodothyronine metabolism and distribution in man by noncompartmental analysis. J. Clin. Endocrinol. Metab 41:319

Okamura, K.,Taurog, A., and Krulich, L. (1981) Hypothyroidism in severely iodine deficient rats. Endocrinology 109:464

Phroah P., Delange F., Fierro- Benitez R, and Stanbury J.B. (1980) Endemic Cretinism In: Endemic Goiter and Endemic Cretinism JB. Stanbury and B.S. Hetzel (eds) John Wiley and Sons, Inc. New York page 395

Riesco, G., Taurog, A., Larsen, P.R., and Krulich, L. (1977) Acute and chronic responses to iodine deficiency in rats. Endocrinology 100:303

Silva, J.E.,Stevenson, C., and Pineda,G. (1973) Plasma iodide concentration, thyroid clearance of plasma iodide and goiter in an area of chronic iodine deficiency. Rev. Med. Chile 101:763

Silva, J.E., (1971) Adaptative mechanisms to iodine deficien cy in man and rat. University of Chile Post Graduate Thesis

Silva, E. (1972) Disposal rates of thyroxine and triiodo-thyronine in iodine deficient rats. Endocrinology 91:1430

Silva, J.E., Pineda, G., and Stevenson, C. (1974) The importance of triiodothyronine as thyroid hormone. In: Endemic Goiter and Cretinism: Continuing threats to world Health. PAHO Sci. Pub #292 page 52

Silva, J.E.,Larsen, P.R. (1978) Contribution of plasma tri-iodothyronine and local thyroxine monodeiodination to to triiodothyronine to nuclear triiodothyronine receptor saturation in pituitary, liver and kidney of hypothyroid rats.Further evidence relating saturation of pituitary nuclear triiodothyronine receptors and the acute inhibition of thyroid stimulating hormone release. J Clin Invest 61:1247

Silva, J.E., Larsen, P.R. (1977) Pituitary nuclear 3,5,3' triiodothyronine and thyrotropin secretion: an explanation for the effect of thyroxine. Science 198:617

Silva, J.E, Dick, T.E., Larsen, P.R. (1978) The contribution of local tissue thyroxine monodeiodination to the nuclear 3,5,3'-triiodothyronine in pituitary, liver and kidney of euthyroid rats. Endocrinology 103:1196

Silva, J.E., and Silva, S. (1981) Interrelationships among serum thyroxine, triiodothyronine, reverse triiodothyronine and thyroid stimulating hormone in iodine-deficient pregnant women and their offspring: effects of iodine supplementation J. Clin Endocrin Metab 52:671

Stevenson,C., Silva, J.E., and Pineda, D. (1974) Thyroxine

and triiodothyronine: Effects of iodine on serum concentration and disposal rates in subjects from an endemic goiter area. J. Clin. Endocrinol. Metab 38:390.

Surks,M.I., Oppenheimer, J.H. (1977) Concentration of L-thyroxine and L-triiodothyronine specifically bound to nuclear receptors in rat liver and kidney; quantitative evidence favoring a major role of T_3 in Thyroid hormone action. J. Clin Invest 60:555

Taurog, A., Porter, J.C., Thio, D.T. (1964) Nature of the 131 I- compounds released into the thyroid veins of rabbits dogs and cats before and after TSH stimulation Endocrinol 74:902

Wayne, E.J., Koutras, D.A., and Alexander, W.D. (1964) Clinical aspects of iodine metabolism. F.A. Davis, Philadelphia,page 3

New Concepts in Thyroid Disease, pages 105–118

MODULATION OF THYROID FUNCTION BY THE SYMPATHETIC NERVOUS SYSTEM

M.A.Pisarev, D.P.Cardinali, M.Barontini, G.J. Juvenal, M.I.Vacas and R.J.Boado
Comisión Nacional de Energía Atómica, Centro de Estudios Farmacológicos y de Principios Naturales, Centro de Investigaciones Endocrinológicas and Laboratorio de Investigaciones Endocrinológicas, Buenos Aires, Argentina.

INTRODUCTION

By classical definition the autonomic nervous system, is that system of motor nerve fibers that supplies the cardiac muscle, smooth muscle (such as that in the blood vessels) and glands, and that consists, in its simplest form, of nerve pathways each comprising two succeding nerve cells. The first neuron is located in the brain or spinal cord and the second in a ganglion, outside the brain and the spinal cord. The location, arrangement, and connection of the two-nerve-cell pathways of the autonomic nervous system form the basis of an anatomical classification or subdivision of the pathways into sympathetic and parasympathetic systems(15).

The superior cervical ganglia (SCG) provide sympathetic innervation to a number of intra and extracranial structures including the pineal gland, cephalic blood vessels, the choroid plexus, the eye, carotid bodies, and the salivary and thyroid glands. Functional alteration of one or many of these structures can be implicated in the neuroendocrine sequelae of superior cervical ganglionectomy (SCGx), which include such disparate effects as the disruption of water balance in pituitary stalk-sectioned rats, the alteration of prolactin release and drinking behavior in rats and the disruption of the photoperiodic controls of reproduction in hamsters, ferrets, voles, rams and goats (for references see ref. nº 6). Although many authors have studied the possible involvement of the sympathetic nervous system in the regulation of thyroid function, there is no general consensus about the sort of influence that catecholamines exert on thyroid cells. Acute iv injection of epinephrine or norepinephrine (NE) to dogs (27) or sheep (12) affected thyroid blood flow without changing labeled hormone secretion. In rabbits, a continuous infusion of epinephrine caused thyroid vasoconstriction as well as depression of the radioiodine uptake (3). A similar decrease in radioiodine uptake was found in rats after epinephrine administration (2). In humans, both stimulatory and inhibitory effects of epinephrine were reported; an acute injection increased ^{131}I uptake, whereas a continuous infusion depressed it (14). In vitro and in vivo experiments have shown that epinephrine and NE can stimulate (17,21-23,32) inhibit (2,20,31) or be devoid of activity on thyroid function (1,11). For example, 6 uM NE added to the incubation medium of thyroid glands inhibited TSH-induced secretion of thyroid hormones (20).

Comparatively less attention has been paid to changes in thyroid activity after surgical or chemical removal of the thyroid gland's sympathetic innervation. Since this sympathetic innervation is known to originate in the SCG it is possible to manipulate the neural input in a number of situations by surgically excising the ganglia or supressing their afferent preganglionic fibers. Sixteen hours after SCGx the endogenous NE stores of the thyroid gland became depleted (Fig.1). Eventually this led, as in other adrenergically innervated organs (35), to an increase in the number of thyroid α-adrenoceptor sites when measured 7 days later (30). The present article reviews recent experiments on the effects of SCGx on various aspects of thyroid function, including the goitrogenic response to methylmercaptoimidazole (MMI) and bovine TSH, ^{131}I uptake, serum TSH, T_3 and T_4 levels, and RNA synthesis. The results obtained suggest that the SCG provide a physiologically relevant input to thyroid cells.

EFFECT OF SCGx ON THE GOITROGENIC RESPONSE

In order to examine the effect of SCGx on the goitrogenic response, rats subjected to surgery 7 days earlier were treated with 4 mg/day of MMI during 4 days and 24 h after the last injection the animals were killed and their thyroids were weighed; plasma TSH concentration

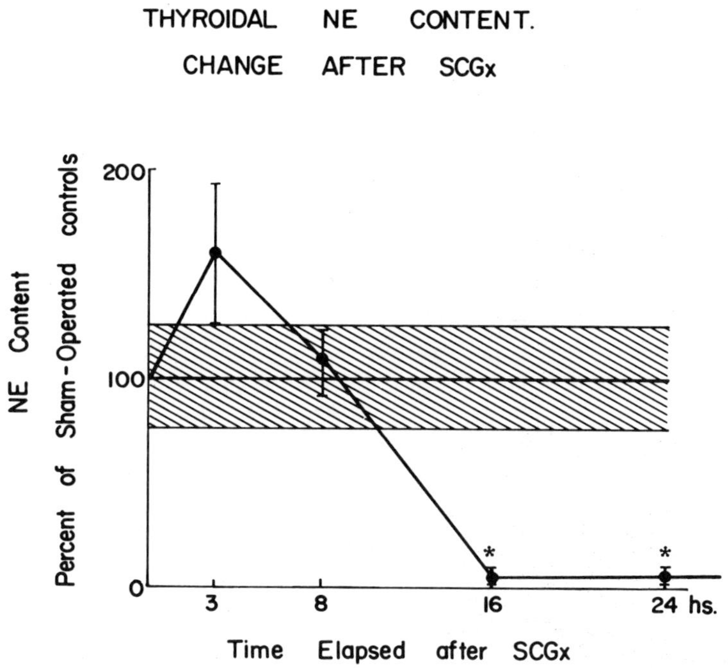

Fig. 1 Male rats were subjected to SCGx or sham-operation and were killed 3-24 h later; NE content was measured by a radio-enzymatic procedure (8). Shown are the means ± SEM (n= 5 to 7 animals/group) of percent control values (NE content in sham operated controls: 396 ± 66 pg/mg thyroid). Asterisks designate significant differences as compared to sham-operated controls ($p < 0.01$, analysis of variance) (Data from ref. nº 5).

was also measured (30). SCGx did not affect any of the parameters studied in saline-injected animals (Fig.2). Factorial analysis (SCGx x MMI) revealed a significant interaction ($p < 0.01$) between MMI and SCGx, i.e. after MMI administration, the increase in thyroid weight was significantly greater in SCGx animals than in sham-operated rats. The plasma TSH responses to MMI treatment were essentially similar in both experimental groups,as

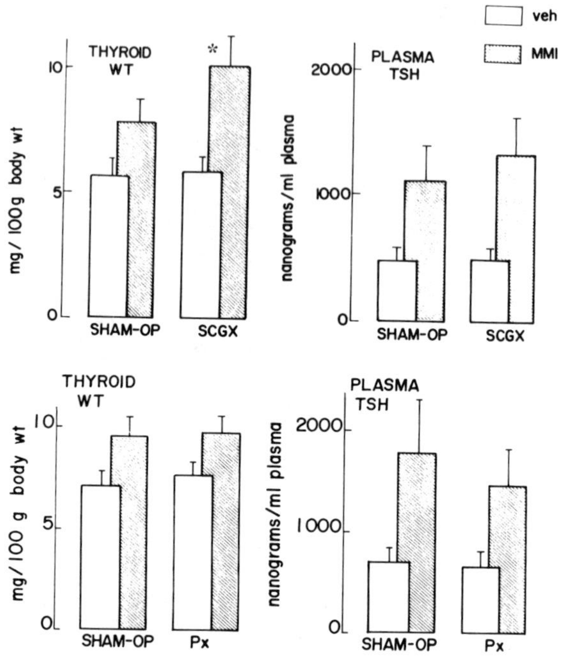

Fig. 2 Effect of SCGx or pinealectomy (Px) on the goitrogenic response to MMI. Male rats subjected to surgery 7 days earlier were injected with MMI (4 mg/day for 4 days). Results are expressed as the mean ± SEM (n= 5 to 7 animals/ group). Rat plasma TSH concentrations were measured by RIA using a double antibody procedure and reagents provided by the Rat Pituitary Hormone Distribution Program (NIAMDD). Results are expressed as nanograms of TSH-RP-1 per ml plasma. The assay sensitivity was 10-20 ng. Statistical analysis was performed by a factorial analysis of variance, followed by a modified t test.(*) $p < 0.05$ (Data from ref.nº 30)

revealed by the absence of the interaction surgery × MMI in the factorial analysis (Fig.2).

As stated above the SCG provides sympathetic innervation to the pineal gland and from the neuroendocrine point of view the importance of this innervation is very conspicuous (26,33). The sympathetic nerve terminals at the pineal gland act by releasing NE which interacts with α- and β-adrenoreceptors on pineal parenchymal cells and activates the synthesis of hormonal products, particularly melatonin (for references see ref. nº 4). Since under certain circumstances, the pineal gland may affect thyroid function via a negative influence exerted either centrally or peripherally at the level of the gland (28,34), the results on ganglia ablation of Fig.2 could be subjected theoretically to any of the following interpretations: 1) SCGx removes a direct inhibitory signal exerted at the thyroid level; 2) SCGx acts indirectly via a functional pinealectomy or 3) SCGx modifies the sensitivity of the thyroid gland to MMI.

A subsequent experiment, in which the goiter induced by MMI in pinealectomized rats was indistinguishable from that found in sham-operated animals (Fig.2), suggested that the pineal gland was not involved in the observed phenomenon (30). A possible central nervous system mechanism affecting TSH release could be also ruled out, since plasma TSH levels were the same in MMI-treated SCGx, or MMI-treated controls rats as well as in MMI-treated pinealectomized, or MMI-treated and sham-pinealectomized rats (Fig.2). In addition, SCGx appeared to exert its progoitrogenic effect even in the absence of MMI, because TSH treatment of denervated rats also resulted in greater than normal thyroid weight compared to similarly treated controls (Fig.3). Seven days after SCG removal, thyroid RNA synthesis increased by 65%, without significant changes in thyroid weight. Eventually spontaneous goiter developed in SCGx rats 4 weeks after surgery (30).

In the rat every thyroid lobe has an ipsilateral sympathetic innervation. This anatomical characteristic allowed us to examine the effect of unilateral SCGx on the spontaneous and MMI- or TSH-induced thyroid growth (Fig.4). Twelve days after removing the right SCG a significantly larger right thyroid lobe, and significantly greater responses to both goitrogenic agents, were observed ($p < 0.05$, paired *t* test). NE content of the right thyroid lobe decreased to about 15-20% of the innervated left lobe after unilateral SCGx (unpublished results).

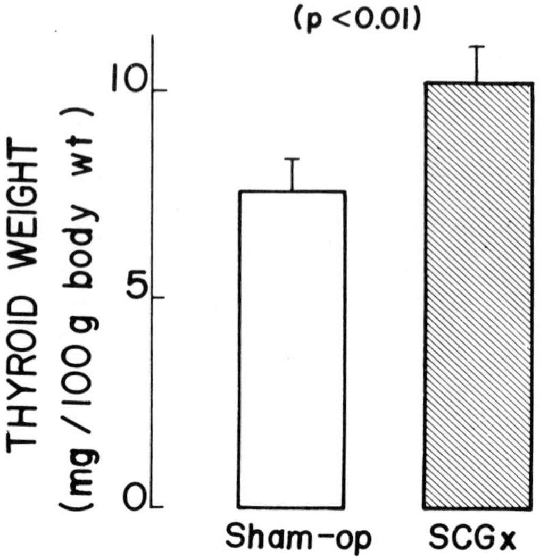

Fig. 3 Effect of SCGx on the goitrogenic response to TSH. Rats subjected to SCGx or sham operation 7 days earlier were injected with TSH (100 mU/day for 4 days). Results are expressed as the mean ± SEM.(n= 8 in each group).The difference between the groups is significant ($p < 0.01$, by Student's <u>t</u> test).(Data from ref. nº 30).

To assess whether SCGx affected thyroid blood flow, we used an iv tracer dose of ^{86}Rb, an accepted method for blood flow estimation (30). Rats subjected to SCGx 7 days earlier exhibited a decreased blood flow, not only in the thyroid gland but also in another sympathetically innervated structure, the pineal gland. A similar decrease in ^{86}Rb uptake by the pineal gland of SCGx rats was reported by Goldman (13). Therefore, our results tended to rule out the conclusion that the removal of the SCG results in changes in blood flow, namely vasodilatation, thereby enhancing the response of the thyroid gland to normal circulating levels of TSH. Rather these data support a direct link of innervation with acini function, probably in the same way other neuroendocrine transducer cells (36). Summarizing, our results support the conclusion that the NE released from the thyroid sympathetic nerves impairs the thyroid response to TSH and that after removal of these postganglionic sympa-

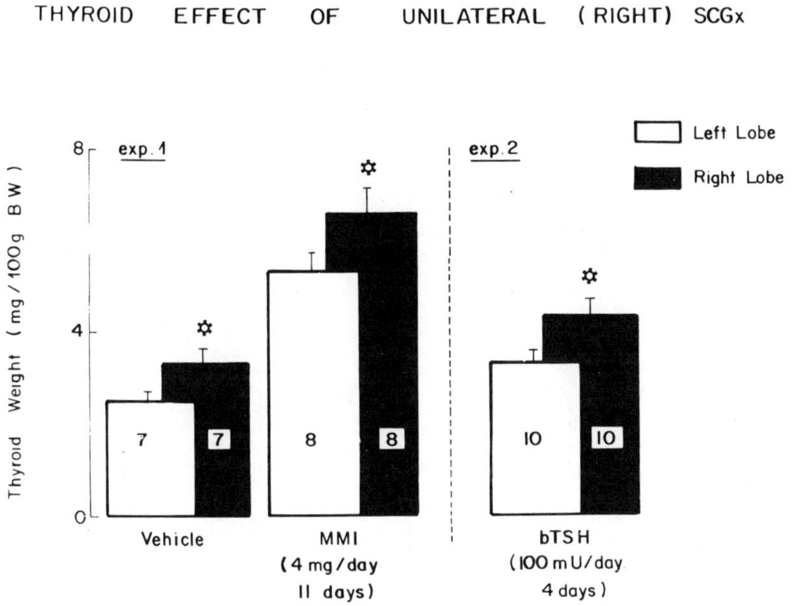

Fig. 4 Rats were subjected to unilateral SCGx and the treatment was started 1 day later (exp 1) or 7 days later (exp 2). (*)p <0.05, paired *t* test.

thetic fibers, stimulation of thyroid growth ensues.The objective of the following series of experiments was to assess the changes in thyroid function at the time of the degeneration of nerve terminals within the gland, shortly after SCGx.

ACUTE EFFECTS OF SCGx ON THE HYPOPHYSIAL-THYROID AXIS

Data from experiments on the nictitating membrane, the salivary glands and the periorbital muscles indicate that after SCGx, and depending upon the length of the axonal stump, a release of NE from varicosities begins at the 10th-14th and elapses for 8-10 h until degeneration of terminals is completed (Fig.1) (10,18). This temporary supraliminal release of neurotransmiter leads to transient hyperactivity of the adrenergically innervated organ and can be a useful procedure to unravel the physiological significance of sympathetic innervation in the regulation of organ's activity. As discussed

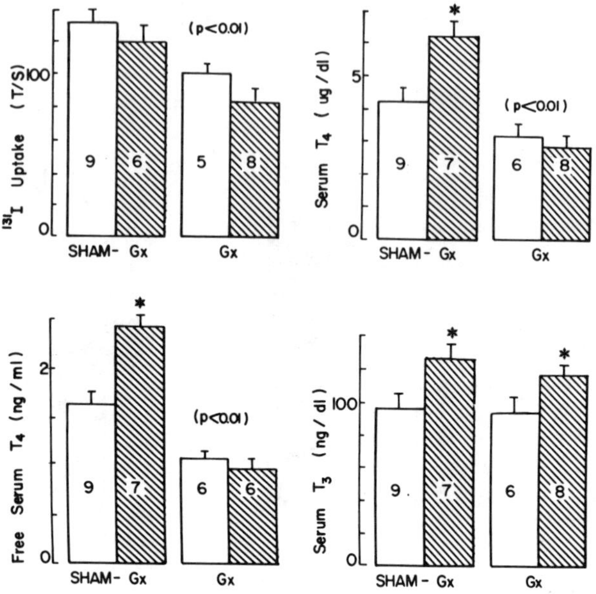

Fig. 5 Rats were subjected to SCGx or sham-operation 14 h earlier and received 250 mU of bovine TSH i.p. (hatched bars) or vehicle (open bars) 1 h before sacrifice. All animals received 80 uCi of ^{131}I i.p. 1 h before sacrifice. Results were analyzed statistically by a factorial analysis of variance followed by a modified t test. As factorial main effects SCGx depressed significantly ^{131}I uptake and total and free serum T_4 ($p < 0.01$) (Data from ref. nº 5).

above in the case of the pituitary-thyroid axis two potential sites of modulatory influence by SCG can be envisioned, i.e. at the level of the thyroid, and centrally on CNS structures that could affect TSH release. The experiment shown in Fig.5 was carried out to assess the changes in the hypophysial-thyroid axis at the time of degeneration of the sympathetic nerves after SCGx (5). A significant depression of total and free T_4 and T_3 was apparent, as well as an impairment in serum T_4 response to exogenous TSH. Likewise circulating TSH decreased by 40-65% 14 h after SCGx (5). These results suggest a depressive effect of acute SCGx on the pitu-

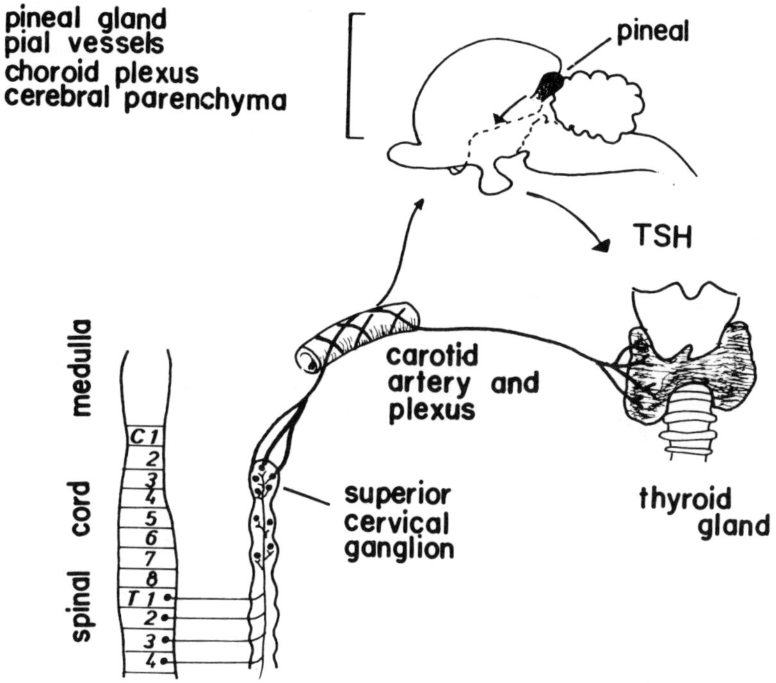

Fig. 6 Territory of the SCG in the rat. The two sites of action (central and peripheral) of sympathetic nerves on thyroid activity are shown.

itary-thyroid axis in rats, exerted both centrally on TSH secretion, and peripherally on the thyroid sensitivity to TSH. They differ from the results depicted in Fig.2 on chronically SCGx animals, in which an impending enhancement of the thyroid response to TSH without changes in serum TSH was observed.

As already stated, the SCG provide sympathetic control of melatonin secretion by the pineal gland (4, 33), provide vasoconstrictor control to brain and pituitary (7,29), and regulate the secretion of the choroid plexus (19) (Fig.6). When SCGx was performed in animals priorly subjected to pineal ablation the central but not the peripheral effect of sympathetic nerve degeneration was observed (5). The SCGx-induced depression of serum TSH was not longer observed in pinealectomized rats although the low serum T_4 levels persisted unchanged. These results strongly suggest that the pineal gland is involved in the regulation of TSH release in the rat.

How the NE released from degenerating nerve terminals in the thyroid modifies the sensitivity of thyroid cells to TSH remains unsolved. These effects could be exerted on the thyroid acini themselves or be secondary to the vascular changes brought about by endogenous catecholamine release. In this sense ^{86}Rb uptake is significantly depressed 14 h after acute SCGx in rats (5). Additionally our present results do not allow us any conclusion as to how NE acts on thyroid cells in the absence of endogenous TSH. It has been reported that in mice injected with high doses of thyroxine (in order to block TSH secretion) NE or E injection increased the number of colloid droplets and the release of radioiodine by thyroid gland (25); a similar effect was observed after unilateral stimulation of SCG or shortly after the injection of 6-hydroxydopamine. Although these observations argue in favor of a stimulating role of catecholamines in the absence of endogenous TSH caution is required in their interpretation since thyroxine treatment may affect the thyroid itself (17) or the sympathetic nerve terminals (9). As mentioned above depending upon the animal species tested as well as on the experimental approach used, in vitro catecholamines have been reported to stimulate, inhibit or be devoid of activity on thyroid function.

CONCLUDING REMARKS

The experiments discussed herein indicate that the SCG influences thyroid function by acting at two different levels, i.e. centrally by affecting TSH release, and locally by altering the sensitivity of thyroid acini to TSH. The central effect of SCGx is restricted to the period of degeneration of nerve terminals and is not longer observed after destruction of the terminals is completed. In contrast the peripheral effect of SCGx does not become compensated (in spite of an impending α-adrenergic supersensitivity as judged by the increase in α-adrenoceptor sites) and leads eventually to a spontaneous goiter. Collectively these data are compatible with the view that neural signals originated in the SCG depress the function of the hypophysial-thyroid axis (Fig.6).

An increasing amount of evidence now suggest that the SCG may be peripheral centers of integration of neural and endocrine signals. Besides innervating significant neuroendocrine structures the SCG are active points of concurrency for hormone signals as revealed by their metabolic changes after steroid of pituitary hormone injection, as well as by the ocurrence of putative receptors for some of the hormones in SCG (6).Our present results strengthen this view and suggest that among the efferent neuroendocrine pathways of the SCG, that affecting the pituitary-thyroid axis may be relevant one.

ACKNOWLEDGEMENTS

These studies were supported by grants from the Consejo Nacional de Investigaciones Científicas y Técnicas de la República Argentina.

REFERENCES

1. Ahn CS, Athans JC, Rosenberg IN (1969). Effects of epinephrine and of alteration in glandular blood flow upon thyroid function: studies using thyroid vein cannulation in dogs. Endocrinology 84: 501.
2. Botkin AL, Jensen H (1952). The effect of epinephrine and thyrotropin on thyroid functions in rats. Endocrinology 50: 68.
3. Brown Grant K, Gibson JG (1956). The effect of exogenous and endogenous adrenaline on the uptake of radio-iodine by the thyroid gland of the rabbit. J Physiol 131: 85.
4. Cardinali DP (1981) Melatonin. A mammalian pineal hormone. Endocrine Rev 2: 327.
5. Cardinali DP, Pisarev MA, Barontini M, Juvenal GJ, Boado RJ, Vacas MI (1982). Efferent neuroendocrine pathways of sympathetic superior cervical ganglia. Early depression of the pituitary-thyroid axis after ganglionectomy. Neuroendocrinology in press.
6. Cardinali DP, Vacas MI, Gejman PV (1981). The sympathetic superior cervical ganglia as peripheral neuroendocrine centers. J Neural Transm 52: 1.

7. Cardinali DP, Vacas, MI, Luchelli de Fortis A, Stefano FJE (1981) Superior cervical ganglionectomy depresses norepinephrine uptake, increases the density of α-adrenoceptor sites and induces supersensitivity to adrenergic drugs in rat medial basal hypothalamus. Neuroendocrinology 33: 199.
8. Da Prada M, Zürcher G (1976) Simultaneous radioenzymatic determination of plasma and tissue adrenaline, noradrenaline and dopamine within the femtomole range. Life Sci 19: 1161.
9. Dratman MB (1978) The mechanism of thyroxine action. In Li CH (ed): "Hormonal Proteins and Peptides" Vol 6 New York: Academic Press p 205.
10. Emmelin N, Trendelenburg U (1972) Degeneration activity after parasympathetic or sympathetic denervation. Rev Physiol Biochem Exp Pharmacol 66: 148.
11. Ericsson LE, Melander A, Owman Ch, Sundler F (1970) Endocytosis of thyroglobulin and release of thyroid hormone in mice by catecholamines and 5-hydroxytryptamine. Endocrinology 87: 915.
12. Falconer IR (1967) The effect of adrenaline and noradrenaline on hormone secretion and blood flow from the thyroid vein in sheep with exteriorized thyroids. J Physiol 188: 425.
13. Goldman H (1967) The nervous control of blood flow to the pineal body. Life Sci 6: 2071.
14. Hays MT (1965) Effect of epinephrine on radioiodine uptake by the normal human thyroid. J Clin Endocrinol Metab 25: 465.
15. Hubbard J (ed) (1974) The Peripheral Nervous System. New York: Plenum.
16. Juvenal GJ, Kleiman de Pisarev DL, Crenovich L, Pisarev MA (1978) Role of neurotransmitters, prostaglandins and glucose on precursor incorporation into the RNA of thyroid slices. Acta Endocrinol (Copenh) 87: 776.
17. Juvenal GJ, Pisarev MA, Kleiman de Pisarev DL, Altschule N (1981) Uptake, metabolism and action of triiodothyronine in calf thyroid slices. Mol Cell Endocr 22: 31.
18. Langer SZ (1966) The degeneration contraction of the nictitating membrane in the unanesthesized cat. J Pharmacol Exp Ther 151: 66.
19. Lindvall M, Edvinsson L, Owman C (1978) Sympathetic nervous control of cerebrospinal fluid produc-

tion from the choroid plexus. Science 201: 176.
20. Maayan ML, Debons AF, Krimsky I, Volpert EM, From A, Dawry F, Siclari E (1977) Inhibition of thyrotropin and dibutyryl cyclic AMP-induced secretion of thyroxine and triiodothyronine by catecholamines. Endocrinology 101: 284.
21. Maayan ML, Ingbar SH (1970) Effects of epinephrine on iodine and intermediary metabolism in isolated thyroid cells. Endocrinology 87: 588.
22. Melander A, Nilsson E, Sundler F (1972) Sympathetic activation of thyroid hormone secretion in mice. Endocrinology 90: 194.
23. Melander A, Ranklev E, Sundler F, Wertergren U (1975) Beta$_2$-adrenergic stimulation of thyroid hormone secretion. Endocrinology 97: 332.
24. Melander A, Sundler F (1972) Interactions between catecholamines, 5-hydroxytryptamine and TSH on the secretion of thyroid hormone. Endocrinology 90:188
25. Melander A, Wertergren U, Ericsson LE, Sundler F (1977) Influence of the sympathetic nervous system on the secretion and metabolism of thyroid hormone. Endocrinology 101: 1228.
26. Moore RY (1978) The innervation of the mammalian pineal gland. Prog Reprod Biol 4: 1.
27. Mowbray JF, Peart WS (1960) Effects of noradrenaline and adrenaline on the thyroid. J Physiol 151: 261.
28. Nir I (1978) Non-reproductive systems and the pineal gland. J Neural Transm (Suppl) 13: 225.
29. Owman Ch, Edvinsson L, Falck B, Nielsen KC (1974) Amine metabolism in brain vessels with particular regard to autonomic innervation and blood-brain barrier. In: Cervos-Navarro J (ed) "Pathology of Cerebral Microcirculation" Berlin, Walter de Gruyter, p 184.
30. Pisarev MA, Cardinali DP, Juvenal GJ, Vacas MI, Barontini M, Boado RJ (1981) The role of the sympathetic nervous system in the control of the goitrogenic response in the rat. Endocrinology 109: 2202.
31. Sherwin JR, Mills I (1980) Epinephrine inhibits thyrotropin-stimulate adenosine 3'5' monophosphate accumulation in cat thyroid slice. Endocrinology 106: 28.
32. Spaulding SW, Burrow GN (1975) Beta adrenergic stimulation of cyclic AMP and protein kinase

activity with thyroid. Nature 254: 347.
33. Vacas MI, Keller Sarmiento MI, Pereyra E, Cardinali DP (1982) Early changes in cAMP and melatonin levels of rat pineal gland after superior cervical ganglionectomy. Neuroendocrinology Lett in press.
34. Vriend J, Reiter RJ, Anderson GR (1979) Effects of the pineal and melatonin on thyroid activity of male golden hamsters. Gen Comp Endocrinol 38: 189.
35. Williams LT, Lefkowitz RJ (1978) Receptor Binding Studies in Adrenergic Pharmacology. Raven Press, New York.
36. Wurtman RJ (1973) Biogenic amines and endocrine function. Introduction: neuroendocrine transducers and monoamines. Fed Proc 32: 1769.

New Concepts in Thyroid Disease, pages 119–130

TSH SECRETION AND REGULATION IN ENDEMIC GOITER AND ENDEMIC CRETINISM

Geraldo Medeiros-Neto

Thyroid Laboratory, Hospital das Clínicas, Faculdade de Medicina da Universidade de São Paulo
São Paulo, Brasil

The pathogenic role of TSH in the development of endemic goiter remains uncertain. In regions of severe iodine deficiency, serum TSH levels were variably increased (1-6). Some of the goitrous subjects, however, had TSH levels within the normal range and enhanced sensitivity to TSH may account for their goiters (Bray, G.A., 1968). It is also quite possible that minor TSH elevations might remain undetected with the current radioimmunoassays or that the TSH elevation is transient and falls when an increased thyroid mass which restores hormone levels to normal is achieved.

In an attempt to further delineate the role of TSH in the pathogenesis of goiter, various groups have administered TRH to goitrous subjects. No significant difference in TSH response to synthetic TRH given intravenously was demonstrable between normal subjects and patients with endemic goiter in a study conducted in Italy (Pinchera, A. 1973). However, Medeiros-Neto et al (Medeiros-Neto, G.A., 1975) in Brazil, Lewitus et al (Lewitus, Z., 1973) in Israel, Scriba et al (Scriba, P.C., 1973) in the German Alps, Rothenbuchner et al (Rothenbuchner, 1974) in Greece, and Kochupiallai et al (Kochupiallai, N., 1973) in the Hymalaias found higher TSH levels in goitrous patients as compared to normal controls and observed that the goitrous subjects had significantly higher peak TSH values than normal controls after TRH injection. A likely explanation for the apparently divergent results would be the difference in the dietary iodine intake for the patients studied in various endemic areas. Adams et al (Adams, D.D., 1971) postulated that there is a negative correlation between levels of iodine intake and plasma TSH; thus thyrotropin is increased when iodine intake is decreased below a critical level.Results from our laboratory reported elsewhere (Adams,D.D.,1971) seem to confirm this hypothesis.When the total dietary iodine intake is less than 50 ug/day the mean TSH basal level in the goitrous patients,living in a rural community,was 6.2 ± 3.0 uU/ml (3.0 - 11.0 uU/ml).In the goitrous patients living in the urban area where the iodine content in the food and water is higher(average:150 ug/day) the mean serum TSH basal level was 3.0 ± 1.3 uU/ml (1.0 - 5.0 uU/ml).

We have also compared the TSH response to TRH in the goitrous patients (living in an endemic goiter area) and compared the results with the same stimulation test performed in normal controls,living in the urban aerea of São Paulo.As shown in Table 1 the goitrous subjects had a significant higher TSH response to TRH in spite of normal serum T_4 levels and as expected,elevated serum T_3 concentrations as compared with the normal subjects.

Table 1.Serum T_4,T_3,basal and peak TSH response to TRH in goitrous and normal subjects.(mean and SD)
(Medeiros-Neto et al,1975)

	Nomal (n=10)	Goitrous (n=20)
T_4 (ug/dl)	8.1 ± 1.6	8.7 + 0.3
T_3 (ng/dl)	132 ± 9.8	186 + 38*
TSH basal (uU/ml)	1.3 ± 1.2	6.2 ± 3.0*
TSH peak (uU/ml)	9.8 ± 4.5	31.1± 7.9*

*$p < 0.05$

We have postulated (Medeiros-Neto,G.A.,1975) that this implies that the pituitary-hypothalamic threshold for inhibition of secretion of TSH by circulating thyroid hormones has been reset to have a persistently high secretion of TSH or a higher storage of thyrotropin at pituitary level,even in the presence of normal serum levels of thyroid hormones.In other areas of endemic goiter,however,it was observed a decrease in the serum concentration of T_4 although serum T_3 levels were kept normal or elevated.In these areas Ermans et al (Ermans,A.M. 1980) have shown that serum TSH levels correlate inversely with the serum concentration of T_4 but not with the concentration of serum T_3 (Figure 1).The patients with,few exception were euthyroid.A similar phenomena can be

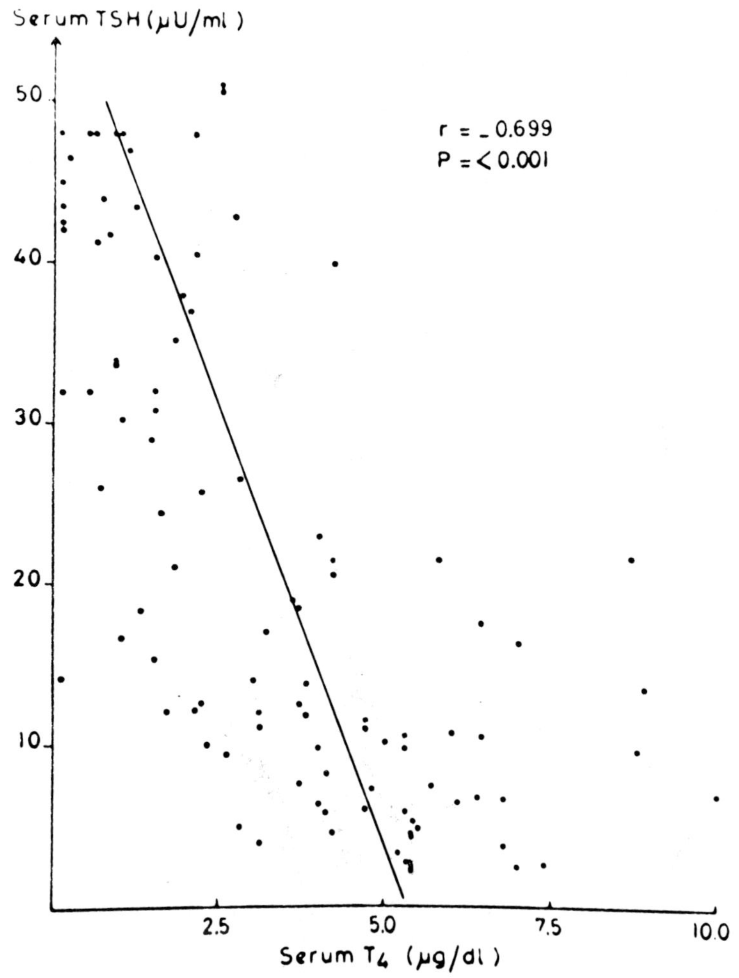

Fig.1-Correlation between serum TSH levels and serum T_4 concentrations.It is shown that TSH has a aignificant negative correlation(r=0.69)with serum T_4 but not with serum T_3(Ermans,1980)

observed in experimental iodine deficiency.When rats are deprived of iodine serum T_4 falls rapidly,serum TSH increases while concentrations remain constant (Fukuda,H.1975).In early studies of this phenomenon it was speculated that the constancy of serum T_3 explained the tendency for the short - term iodine deficient rat to maintain a normal thyroid status even though serum TSH was increased.More recently Larsen et al (Larsen,P.R. 1981)have shown that the ratio of intracellularly produced nuclear $T_3$to plasma T_4 is substantially higher in the pituitary than in the liver or kidney.Therefore in the absence of T_4 the pituitary-nuclear/plasma T_3 ratio does not increase sufficiently to compensate for the lack of intracellular T_4 to T_3 convertion.On the other hand if serum T_3 remains relatively constant(or even high) then nuclear receptor saturation in tissues such as liver and kidney and heart would remain at euthyroid levels.As a consequence of the goitrous individuals can mantain an elevated TSH secretion in the presence of a normal or high serum T_3 and would be hyper-responsive to the TRH stimulation.

Early observations from our laboratory(Meddeiros-Neto, G.A.,1975) have shown that endemic goiter patients when moving to an urban area had a normal serum basal TSH and a normal TSH response to TRH.Studer et al (Studer,H.,1965) also demonstrated a few years ago that iodine defficient rats rapidly corrected the changes in T_4,T_3,and TSH after small iodide loads.Moreover it is common knowledge that iodide supplements given to goitrous subjects in endemic goiter regions may elevate the serum concentration of thyroid hormones,and in some patients,produce hyperthyroidism(so called Jod-Basedow).The basis of this phenomenon are probably autonomus areas in the multinodular goiters.More recently Trost et al (Trost,B.N.,1980) recently demonstrated that a small supplement of 400 ug of iodide per day for 6 days,given to goitrous individuals will significantly reduce the maximal increase of TSH after TRH without significantly changing serum T_3 or T_4.We have decided to study,therefore what would be the natural course of thyroid and pituitary-thyroid relationship in 23 goitrous patients that immigrated to an urban aerea where iodide supply is more abundant ($>$150 ug/day) than in the local endemic goiter aerea ($<$ 50 ug iodide/day).In Figure 2 it is shown that after 3-6 weeks of additional iodide supplementation 7 patients developed a typicalJod-Basedow syndrome.Both T_4 and T_3 were elevated above the normal range,there were a few clinical signs of thyrotoxicosis and TSH response to TRH was blunted.

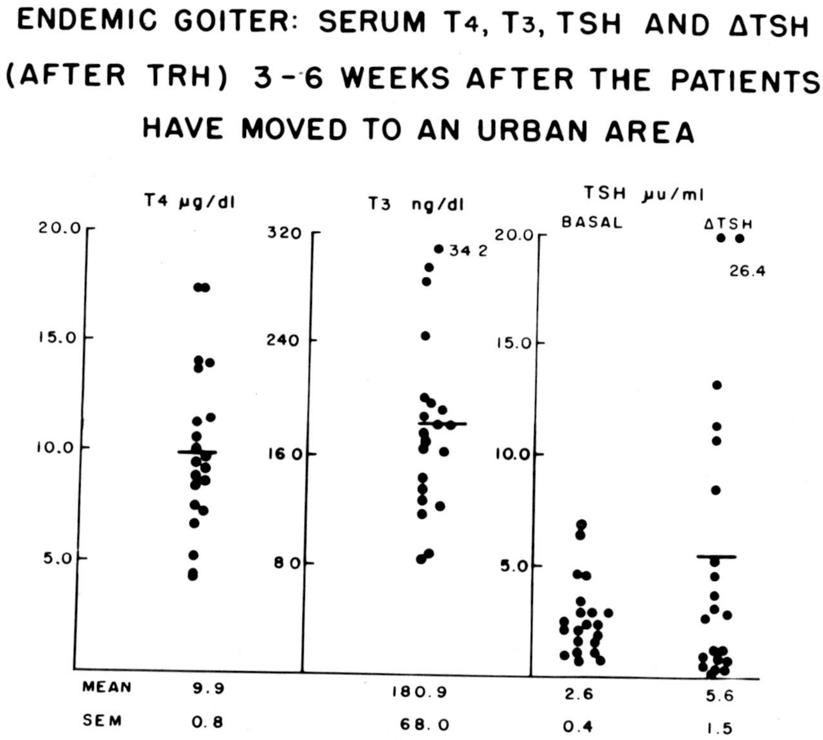

Fig.2-Serum T_4,T_3,and peak TSH response to TRH in 23 goiter patients that immigrated from rural villages (< 50 ugI/day) to an urban community (> 150 ugI/day).Note that 3-6 weeks after being exposed to a higher iodine intake 7 patients became hyperthyroid and 15 additional subjects had a blunted TSH response toTRH.

Fifteen euthyroid goitrous patients had a blunted TSH response to TRH although serum T_3 or T_4 were within the normal range.Only two patients had a typical exaggerated TSH response to TRH,as commonly observed in the endemic goiter aerea.Urinary excretions of iodide was measured in every patient and was in the range of 150-450 ug of iodide/g of creatinine.Therefore these patients were receiving an iodide load through the iodized salt and industrialized food comparable to the iodide supplementation given experimentally by Trost et al (Trost,B.N.,1980) to normal and goitrous subjects. The explanation for the Jod-Basedow phenomenon is reasonably clear: these patients, most probably have autonomus nodules that produce a significantly higher level of both T_3 and T_4 in face of an iodide load. The blunted TSH response to TRH, however, in the presence of normal concentrations of both T_3 and T_4 is not easily understandable.

In some of the goitrous patients studied by Trost et al (Trost,B.N.,1980) there was a significant increase in the serum concentrations of both T_3 and T_4, followed by a blunted TSH response to TRH after only 6 days of the small iodide load administered in their experimental design. It is possible that a transient surge of both thyroid hormones would accelerate the intra-pituitary conversion of T_4 to T_3 and saturate the pituitary nuclear receptors, inducing a block in TSH synthesis and release, when the endemic thyroid gland is receiving more iodide.

Endemic Cretinism

In addition to the extreme types of endemic cretinism, corresponding, respectively to the neurologic and myxedematous cretins, there exists a continuous spectrum of abnormalities of development, reflecting different degrees of impairment in the nervous system and in thyroid function. We have previously reported discrete signs of thyroid insufficiency in the so called neurological cretins in agreement with this concept (Medeiros-Neto,G.A.,1978). At present the crucial problem posed by endemic cretinism is its ethiopathogenis and the mechanisms responsible for different manifestations in many parts of the world. Its most likely cause is thought to be a defective maduration of the central nervous system during the critical period covering the end of fetal life and the first months after birth, secondary to an unsufficient level of thyroid hormones or of iodine "per se" (Thilly,C.H., 1974). It seems probable that thyroid insufficiency detected at birth in endemic goiter areas exists also during fetal life. Recovery of adequate thyroid function during the first months of post-natal life is probably complicated by the low iodine content of maternal milk. Thilly et al (Thilly,C.H., 1974 were able to demonstrate that newborns from mothers that did not receive iodide supplementation (iodized oil) during pregnancy have a significantly higher cord-blood level of TSH (26 ng/ml) as compared with the newborns of mothers treated with iodized oil (4.5 ng/ml). More than half of the newborns in the untreated group had levels of T_4 and TSH in the same ranges as those found in the myxedematous cretins and a negative correlation between cord serum T_4 and TSH (r=0.53)was observed.These results demonstrate that a high percentage of newborns in an area of severe endemic goiter have thyroid insufficiency and marked thyrotropic stimulation.At this point most of these infants will adapt to the chronic iodine deficiency and the increased TSH levels would stimulate the thyroid gland to a marked hyperplasia.A small number of the children born in the endemic area,however,will fail to adapt to the iodine deficiency and would present,pesistently,clinical and laboratory hyperthyroidism.

In other regions of chronic iodine deficiency,however, a subclinical hypothyroidism is usually present in the neurological cretins.In spite of normal levels of T_4 and T_3 these patients have an exaggerated and sustained TSH response to TRH (Trost,B.N.,1980) and are extremely sensitive to an iodide load,which rapidily induces a full clinical picture of hypothyroidism.

We have studied,recently,a group of 27 patients with long standing untreated endemic cretinism living in an isolated village in Central Brazil (Medeiros-Neto,G.A.,1980). The patients were clinically divided into three groups: Hypothyroid (Pinchera,A.,1973),goitrous cretins clinically euthyroid (Adams,D.D. 1971) and five cretins without goiter. The 27 patients in this study had serum concentration of T_4, T_3,TSH,alpha subunit and TSH-beta and Prolactin measured before and after a TRH test.Fourteen patients also had a lateral skull film performed to evaluate the size of the sella turcica.In seven of the hypothyroid endemic cretins there was a marked enlargement of the sella turcica with cortical bone thinning and erosion in addition to balooning of the sella (Medeiros-Neto,G.A.,1981).The mean TSH level was markedly elevated at 46 $\pm$ 24 uU/ml as was the peak TSH response of 118 $\pm$ 42 uU/ml 30 min after TRH administration. The pituitary enlargement was probably secondary to the long standing untreated thyroid failure.These hypothyroid subjects also showed the largest alpha sub unit response to TRH (1.7 $\pm$ 0.3 to 3.4$\pm$ 0.9 ng/ml)as shown in Figure 3. Although the mean basal (2.3 $\pm$ 0.5 uU/ml)and TRH stimulated (20 $\pm$ 4.7 uU/ml) TSH levels in the neurological goitrous cretins were normal,5 patients showed increased TSH responses after TRH (Figure 4).Similarly three of the five cretins

ALPHA SUBUNIT RESPONSE TO TRH IN ENDEMIC CRETINISM

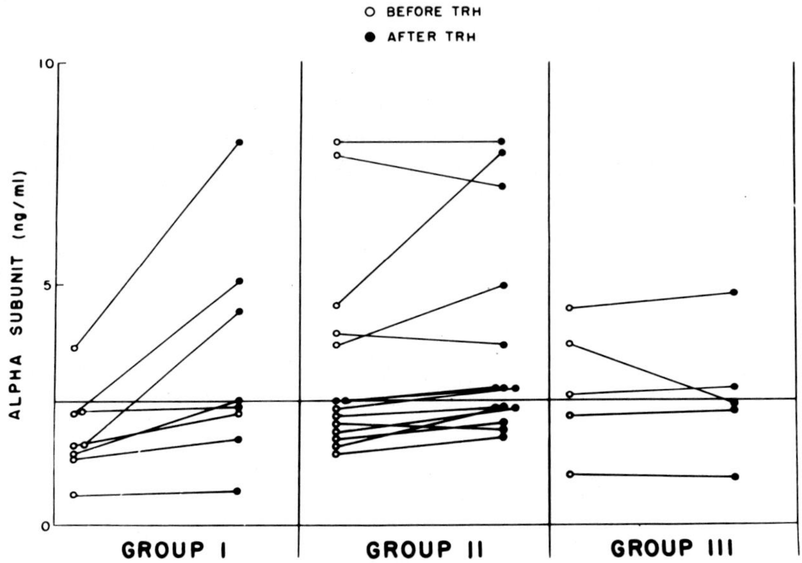

TSH - BETA SUBUNIT RESPONSE TO TRH IN ENDEMIC CRETINISM

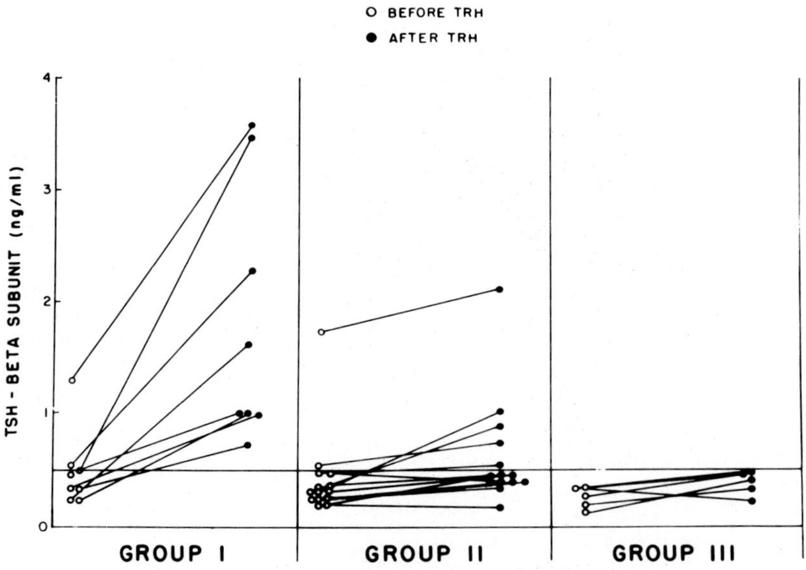

Fig.3-Alpha sub unit and TSH-beta,before and after TRH in hypothyroid(group I) and neurologic (groups II and III) endemic cretins.These patients have a higher than normal alpha sub unit response to TRH and an enlargement of the sella turcica,but this was not considered as suggestive of a pituitary tumour(Medeiros-Neto et al,1980)

without goiter had an elevated TRH-stimulated TSH level. Alpha subunit and TSH levels and TRH stimulated were appropriate for age and sex of these two groups of patients. We have provided evidence,therefore for the concept that thyrotropin cell function is augmented with increased TSH, alpha and TSH beta secretion in long standing myxedematous cretins but not with the neurological type of endemic cretinism.However,the patients in this latter category may have a decreased thyroid reserve,as defined by an exaggerated TSH response to TRH and would eventually become hypothyroid later in adult life.

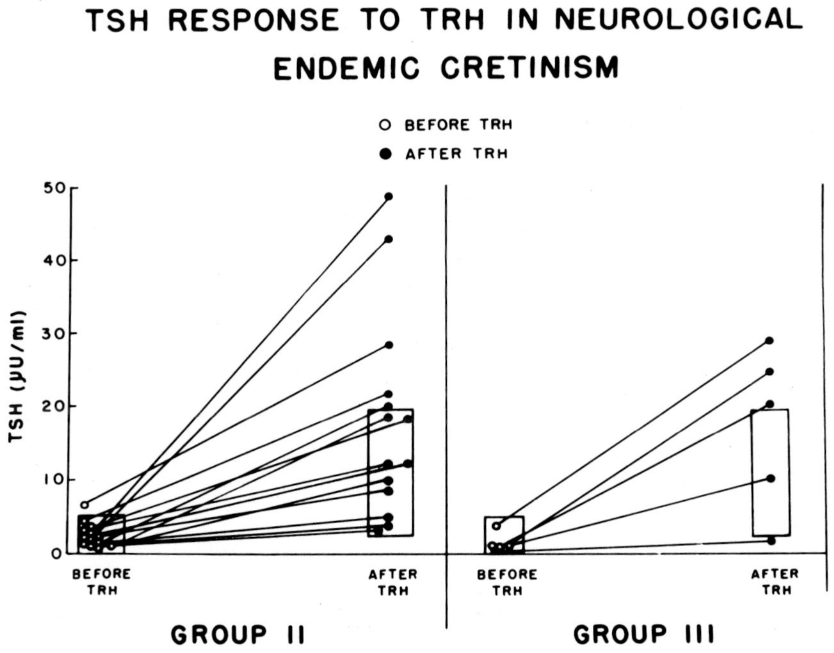

Fig.4-Neurological euthyroid endemic cretins may have an exaggerated TSH response to TRH indicating impeding thyroid failure (Medeiros-Neto et al,1980)

Abstract

In endemic goiter patients living in a chronic iodide deficiency area ($<$ 50ug/day) TSH basal levels and the TSH response to TRH is significantly higher(31 $\pm$ 8uU/ml) than in normal controls (10 $\pm$ 4uU/ml).There is a negative co-rrelation between levels of iodine intake and serum TSH concentration and thyrotropin is thus increased when iodine dicreased . Also it was shown that serumTSH levels correlate inversely with the serum concentration of T_4 (r=0.69) but not with the usually normal or elevated serum concentration of T_3 in endemic goiter patients.It has been postulated that in the absence of appropriate serum levels of T_4 the pituitary thyrotrophs have an abnormally low T_4 to T_3 conversion and the pituitary-nuclear/serum T_3 ratio does not increase sufficiently to compensate this phenomenon.On the other hand nuclear receptor saturation of T_3 in tissues such as liver and kidney would remain at euthyroid levels due to the higher serum T_3 concentrations.Endemic goiter patients when moving to an urban area where iodine intake is higher ($>$150ug/day) than in the rural villages,had a blunted TSH response to TRH (15/23 subjects) or developed a mild clinical and laboratory picture of hyperthyroidism (7/23 individuals).Serum TSH levels and the TSH response to TRH is abnormally elevated in the myxedematous type of endemic cretinism but more than one third of the neurological goitrous cretins (euthyroid) have an exaggerated and sustained TSH response to TRH.This has been considered as a decreased thyroid reserve.Measurement of alpha subunits and TSH-beta in both types of endemic cretinism demonstrated that although these patients have a marked enlargement of the sella turcica the alpha subunits,although higher than normal (1.7-3.4 ng/ml)were not suggestive of a pituitary tumour. The pituitary enlargement was probably secondary to the long standing untreated thyroid failure.

REFERENCES

Adams,D.D.,Kennedy,T.H.,Utiger,R.D.,1971 Serm TSH concentrations:measurements by bioassay and immunoassay in iodine deficiency and other states,in:Fellinger,K. and Höfer,R. eds."Further advances in Thyroid Research" Wiener Med Akad, Vienna,p.1044

Bray,G.A.,1968 Increased sensitivity of the thyroid in iodine-depleted rats to the goitrogenic effects of TSH J Clin Investig 47:1640

Buttfield,I.H.,Hetzek,B.S.,Odell,W.O.,1968 Effects of iodized oil on serum TSH determined by immunoassay in endemic goiter subjects J Clin Endocrinol Metab 28:1664

Coble,Y.D.,Kobler,P.O.,1970 Plasma TSH levels in endemic goiter subjects J Clin Endocrinol Metab 31:220

Delange,F.,Hershman,J.M.,Ermans,A.M.,1971 Relationship between the serum TSH level,the prevalence of goiter and the pattern of iodine metabolism in Idjwi Island J Clin Endocrinol Metab 33:261

Ermans,A.M.,1980 Ethiopathogenesis of Endemic Goiter in: Stanbury,J.B. and Hetzel,B.S."Endemic Goiter and Endemic Cretinism" J.Wiley & Sons,New York p.287

Fukuda,H.,Yasuda,N.,Greer,M.A.,Kutas,M and Greer,S.E.,1975 Changes in plasma thyroxine,T_3 and TSH during adaptation to iodine deficiency Endocrinology 97:307

Kovhupillai,N.,Karmakar,M.C.,Weightman,D.,Hall,R.,Deo,M.G., McKendrik,M.,Evered,D.C. and Ramalingaswami,V. et al,1973 Pituitary-thyroid axis in Hymalayan endemic goiter LANCET 1:1021

Larsen,P.R.,Silva,J.E. and Kaplan,M.M.,1981 Relationship between circulating and intracellular thyroid hormones: physiological and clinical implications Endocrine Reviews 2:87

Lewitus,Z.,Rechnic,J.and Laor,J.,1973 TSH response to TRH in an endemic goiter area in Israel Acta Endocrinol Suppl 179:49

Medeiros-Neto,G.A.,Penna,M.,Monteiro,K.,Kataoka,K.,Imai,Y. and Hollander,C.S.,1975 The effect of iodized oil in the TSH response to TRH in endemic goiter patients J Clin Endocrinol Metab 41:504

Medeiros-Neto,G.A.,Hollander,C.S.,Knobel,M.,Imai,I.and Kataoka,K. Effects of iodides on the hypothalamic-pituitary-thyroid axis in neurological endemic cretinism:evidence for compensated thyroidal failure in adult life.Clin Endocr 8:213

Medeiros-Neto,G.A.,Cavaliere,H.,Almeida,F,Gomes,E.and Kourides,I.A. 1980 Pituitary-thyroid relationship in endemic cretinism:results of T_3,TSH,alpha and TSH-Beta subunits responses to TRH in :Albertini,A."Radioimmunoassay of hormones,proteins and enzynes",Excerpta Medica ICS 528:83

Medeiros-Neto,G.A.,Kourides,I.A.,Almeida,F. and Ingbar,S.H. 1981 Enlargement of the sella turcica in some patients long-standing untreated endemic cretinism.Serum TSH,alpha, TSH-beta and prolactin responses to TRH J Endocrinol Investig 4:xxx(in press)

Ogihara,T.,Yamamoto,T.,Fukuchi,M.and Ari,K. 1972 Serum TSH levels of natives in Sarawak,Borneo J Clin Endocrinol Metab 35:711

Pisarev,M.A.,Utiger,R.D.,Salvaneschi,J.P.1970 Serum TSH and thyroxine in goitrous subjects in Argentina J Clin Endocrinol Metab 30:680

Pinchera,A.,Martino,E,Loi,A.M. 1973 TSH response to TRH in endemic goiter Acta Endocrinol Suppl 179:84

Rothenbuchner,G.,Koutras,D.A.,Raptis,S.,Berk,J.,Loos,U. Rigopoulos.G. and Malamos,B. 1974 The effect of TRH on serum TSH levels in non-toxic goiter Horm Metab Res 6:501

Scriba,P.C.,Borowzak,H,Erbardt,F. 1973 Serum gesamt T_3 spiegel und TSH-Reaktion auf TRH-stimulation beim endemischen kropf Acta Endocrinol Suppl 179:53

Studer,H&Greer,M.A. 1965 A study of the mechanism involved in the production of iodine-deficiency goiter Acta Endocrinol 49:610

Thilly,C.H.,Delange,F.Camus,M.,Berquist,H. and Ermans,A.M. 1974 Fetal hypothyroidism in endemic goiter in:Dunn,J.T. & Medeiros-Neto,G.A. "Endemic Goiter and Cretinism: continuing threats to world Health"

Trost,B.N.,Buchli,R.,Osterwälder,H.J.,Kohler,H.,Koenig,M.P. and Studer,H. 1980 The handling of moderately excessive iodide loads by normal and goitrous human thyroid glands J.Molec.Med.4:167

Wahner,W.H.,Mayberry,W.E.,Gaitan,E. 1971 Endemic goiter in the Cauca Valley:role of serum TSH in goitrogenesis. J Clin Endocrinol Metab 32:491

New Concepts in Thyroid Disease, pages 131–137

CONTROL OF THYROTROPIN SECRETION BY THYROXINE AND TRIIODOTHYRONINE

Rubén Boado, Edgardo Ulloa and Angel A. Zaninovich.
Endocrine Research Laboratory (PLABIEN), CONICET, Center of Nuclear Medicine, Hospital de Clínicas José de San Martín, 1453 Buenos Aires, Argentina.

It has long been known that thyroxine (T4) and triiodothyronine (T3) exert a negative feedback effect on the pituitary thyrotropin (TSH) secretion, opposite to the stimulatory effect of the TSH-releasing hormone (TRH). However, the demonstration that T4 converts to T3 in man (Braverman et al. 1970) and in the rat (Schwartz et al. 1971) has led to the suggestion that T3 is the active thyroid hormone (Oppenheimer et al. 1974) leaving for T4 the role of a prohormone. This postulation gained credence by the findings of specific receptor sites for T3 in cell nucleus of several tissues of experimental animals (Oppenheimer et al. 1974, Samuels & Tsai 1974, DeGroot & Torresani 1975). Such nuclear sites can also bind T4 albeit with a lower affinity. In the last few years many groups of investigators have studied the effects of thyroid hormones on the secretion of TSH as a model for hormone action. Fukuda, Yasuda & Greer (1975) have studied the effects of equiphysiological doses of T4 and T3 on the TSH secretion in normal and low iodine-treated rats. The administration of 1 ug of T4/100 g BW or 250 ng of T3/100 g BW, induced a rapid fall in serum TSH concentration within 15 minutes, and became significant one hour after the injection. However, the study did not assess the conversion of T4 to T3 in the tissues. Recently, Connors & Hedge (1981) studied the effect of a continuous infusion of 1 or 2 ug of T4/100 g BW or 280 ng of T3/100 g BW/day during 96 hours to thyroidectomized rats. In these experiments 2 ug of T4/100 g significantly reduced the TSH response to TRH and 1 ug of T4 or 280 ng of T3/100 g produced no changes in serum TSH 10 minutes after TRH. In animals treated with 2 ug of T4/100 g the serum T3 concentration averaged 20 ng/dl similar to the T3 -treated rats. These results show that serum T4 is capable of directly inhibiting the secretion of TSH. Previous work of Silva & Larsen (1977) also showed that T4 can inhibit the release of TSH before its conversion to T3 in hypothyroid rats. However, based on studies of Grimberg et al. (1963), these authors demonstrated that 1 hour after the injection of T4 to hypothyroid rats only T3 could be found in nuclei of pituitary cells and in similar concentrations to those found after the administration of T3. These findings led the authors to suggest that the T3 generated by intrapituitary conversion of T4 was responsible for the control of TSH secretion (Silva & Larsen 1977). This view was supported by further investigations of these (Larsen et al. 1979) and other authors (Obregon et al. 1980).

In our laboratory, we studied the effects of T4 and T3 on the TSH response to TRH and the intrapituitary conversion of T4 to T3 within 30 minutes after T4 administration in normal and iopanoic acid (IOP)-treated rats (Boado et al. 1982a). A group of euthyroid male rats was injected a single iv dose of 6 ug of T4/100 g BW, 1 ug of T3/100 g BW or saline. Twenty minutes later 1 ug of TRH/100 g BW was administered iv. Heparinized blood samples were drawn at time zero (preceding the injection of T4, T3 or saline), at 20 minutes (preceding the injection of TRH) and at 30 minutes (10 minutes post-TRH). In our experience and that of other authors (Lifschitz et al. 1978) this dose and timing of the TRH test adequately reflected the maximal TSH response. Other groups of animals were treated with intraperitoneal injections of IOP (5 mg/100 g BW) every 12 hours starting 48 hours before the initiation of the study in order to prevent the conversion of T4 to T3 (Larsen et al. 1979, Kaplan 1980, Obregon et al. 1980). Thereafter, they received iv 1 or 6 ug of T4/100 g BW, 0.21 or 2.5 ug of T3/100 g BW or saline. TRH test was performed as described

Table 1. Effects of T4 and T3 on the TSH response to TRH in normal and IOP-treated rats[1]. Mean value ± SEM.

Plasma TSH 10 min post-TRH % of control[2]	Plasma T4 Basal ug/dl	Plasma T4 20 min[3] % basal	Plasma T3 Basal ng/dl	Plasma T3 20 min[3] % basal	Pituitary T3 pg
		T4 6 ug/100 g BW (6)[4]			
59[5] ±10	3.1 ±0.3	1503 ±188	142 ±8	66 ±10	16 ±5
		T3 1 ug/100 g BW (6)			
118 ±7	4.2 ±0.2	123 ±4	102 ±10	356 ±109	60 ±10
		T4 1 ug/100 g BW + IOP (7)			
93 ±15	4.0 ±0.3	232 ±24	80 ±5	98 ±9	1.5 ±0.5
		T4 6 ug/100 g BW + IOP (8)			
56[5] ±7	6.6 ±0.8	684 ±76	58 ±10	113 ±12	9 ±3
		T3 0.21 ug/100 g BW + IOP (10)			
111 ±14	2.7 ±0.4	125 ±5	77 ±6	195 ±4	13 ±2
		T3 2.5 ug/100 g BW + IOP (14)			
62[5] ±8	5.5 ±0.8	124 ±7	104 ±17	1454 ±283	150 ±25

1 A dose of 1 ug TRH/100 g BW was injected iv 20 minutes after the iv administration of T4, T3 or saline.
2 Compares TSH response to TRH between experimental and control groups.
3 Blood drawn immediately prior to the administration of TRH
4 Number of experiments.
5 $p < 0.01$ versus control group.

above. Plasma TSH (NIAMDD-kit), T4 and T3 were measured by radioimmunoassay using methods described previously (Boado et al. 1982b, Chopra 1972). Table 1 shows the results obtained. In rats treated with 6 ug of T4/100 g BW the post-TRH increment was 59 %

of the control group ($p < 0.01$). Animals treated with 1 ug of T3/100 g BW had a normal response compared to the effect of saline alone. In rats with depressed intrapituitary conversion of T4 to T3 due to IOP treatment, the injection of 0.21 ug of T3 or 1 ug of T4/100 g BW elicited a normal response to TRH comparing to control IOP-treated rats. When the dose of T4 was increased to 6 ug/100 g the pituitary response to TRH was significantly smaller than in the control group ($p < 0.01$), while plasma T4 was elevated and plasma T3 was within the normal range. In IOP-treated animals injected with 2.5 ug of T3/100 g BW the TSH response to TRH decreased significantly from control values ($p < 0.01$). The degree of conversion of T4 to T3 within the hypophysis during 30 minutes after the injection of T4 was studied by a radiochromatographic technique described previously (Silva & Larsen 1977, Obregon et al. 1980, Boado et al. 1982a). ^{125}I-T4 was prepared by ^{125}I iodination of 3,5-diiodothyronine using a method of Kochupillai & Yallow (1978). Other rats were injected with ^{125}I-T3 and killed 30 minutes later for determination of pituitary ^{125}I-T3. Chromatography of extracted pituitary homogenates from rats not given IOP and injected with ^{125}I-T4 showed that at 30 minutes 5.6×10^{-3} % of the injected radioactivity was due to ^{125}I-T4, 0.25×10^{-3} % ^{125}I-T3 and 0.04×10^{-3} % due to $^{125}I^{-}$. In rats treated with IOP the respective values at 30 minutes post ^{125}I-T4 injection were 6.1 ^{125}I-T4, 0.13 ^{125}I-T3 and 0.1 $^{125}I^{-} \times 10^{-3}$ % respectively. The mean intrapituitary radioactivity due to ^{125}I-T3 30 minutes after the iv injection of ^{125}I-T3 was 6.0 % of the injected dose $\times 10^{-3}$.

The present in vivo data was obtained in euthyroid rats, therefore having a physiological sensitivity of the TSH secreting mechanisms to stimulation by TRH or depression by thyroid hormones. The animals with IOP-induced depressed conversion of T4 to T3 had a significantly decreased TSH response to TRH 30 minutes after the T4 injection, with a decline in TSH levels similar to those obtained with a physiologically equivalent amount of T3. This observation gained relevance by the fact that the calculated amount of intrapituitary T3 generated from T4 conversion at 30 minutes plus the T3 contaminating the injected T4 solution was 9 pg (see Table 1). This quantity of T3 is smaller than the 13 pg present in the hypophysis 30 minutes after the iv injection of 0.21 ug of T3, amount which given to IOP-treated rats failed to depress the TSH response to TRH. Moreover, in rats not receiving IOP and therefore with normal conversion of T4 to T3, the administration of 6 ug of T4 could give rise by intrapituitary conversion at 30 minutes a calculated maximum of 16 pg of T3 (see Table 1); this represents one-third of the intrapituitary T3 in rats injected 1 ug of T3 iv and showing a normal response to TRH. Although T4 analogues may also bind to nuclear pituitary receptors, T4 is the hormone present in the hypophysis for hormone action and conversion to T3. The results displayed here indicate that T4 seems to possess intrinsic hormonal capacity to regulate the secretion of TSH in response to TRH. This conclusion is in accord with previous findings reported by Chopra et al. (1978). These authors observed that in the rat T4 inhibited the TSH response to TRH in vitro in the absence of measurable T3 both in the pituitary and the suspending medium, hence reflecting that T4 per se was responsible for that effect. The studies in humans indicate that serum TSH levels have often been seen to be more related to serum T4 than to serum T3 concentration (Chopra et al. 1975, Klein et al. 1976, Silva & Silva 1981). Perhaps, as suggested by Chopra (1981) T4 conversion to T3 serves to derive T4 maximal biological effects, though T4 appears to be able to exert hormonal activity when its conversion to T3 does not occur.

REFERENCES

Boado R, Ulloa E, Zaninovich AA (1982a). The effects of thyroxine and triiodothyronine on the thyrotropin response to thyrotropin-releasing hormone in normal and iopanoic acid-treated euthyroid rats. Acta Endocrinol (Copenh) 101: in press.

Boado R, Ulloa E, Zaninovich AA (1982b). Reciprocal effects of an acute load of thyroxine or triiodothyronine on their peripheral metabolism and deiodination in the cold-acclimated rat. J Endocrinol Invest in press.

Braverman LE, Ingbar SH, Sterling K (1970). Conver-

sion of thyroxine (T4) to triiodothyronine (T3) in athyreotic human subjects. J Clin Invest 49:855.
Chopra IJ (1972). A radioimmunoassay for measurement of thyroxine in unextracted serum. J Clin Endocrinol Metab 34:938.
Chopra IJ (1981). New insights into metabolism of thyroid hormones: physiological and clinical implications. In Soto RJ, De Nicola A, Blaquier J (eds): "Physiopathology of Endocrine Diseases and Mechanism of Hormone Action," New York: Alan R. Liss, p 67.
Chopra IJ, Carlson HE, Solomon DH (1978). Comparison of inhibitory effects of 3,5,3'-triiodothyronine (T3), thyroxine (T4), 3,3',5'-triiodothyronine (rT3) and 3,3'-diiodothyronine (T2) on thyrotropin-releasing hormone-induced release of thyrotropin in the rat in vitro. Endocrinology 103:393.
Chopra IJ, Hershman JM, Hornabrook RW (1975). Serum thyroid hormone and thyrotropin levels in subjects from endemic goiter regions of New Guinea. J Clin Endocrinol Metab 40:326.
Connors JM, Hedge GA (1981). Effect of continuous thyroxine administration on thyrotropin secretion in thyroidectomized rats. Endocrinology 108:2098.
DeGroot LJ, Torresani J (1975). Triiodothyronine binding to isolated liver cell nuclei. Endocrinology 96:357.
Fukuda H, Yasuda H, Greer MA (1975). Acute effects of thyroxine, triiodothyronine and iodide on thyrotropin secretion. Endocrinology 97:924.
Grimberg R, Volpert EM, Werner SC (1963). In vivo deiodination of labeled L-thyroxine to 3,5,3'-triiodothyronine in mouse and human pituitaries. J Clin Endocrinol Metab 23:140.
Kaplan MM (1980). Thyroxine 5'-monodeiodination in rat anterior pituitary homogenates. Endocrinology 106:567.
Klein AH, Foley Jr TP, Larsen PR, Agustin AV, Hopwood NJ (1976). Neonatal thyroid function in congenital hypothyroidism. J Pediat 89:545.
Kochupillai N, Yallow RS (1978). Preparation, purification and stability of high specific activity ^{125}I-labeled thyronines. Endocrinology 102:128.
Larsen PR, Dick TE, Markovitz BP, Kaplan MM, Gard T G (1979). Inhibition of intrapituitary thyroxine to 3,5,3'-triiodothyronine conversion prevents the acute suppression of thyrotropin release by thyro-

xine in hypothyroid rats. J Clin Invest 64:117.
Lifschitz BM, Defesi CR, Surks MI (1978). Thyrotropin response to thyrotropin-releasing hormone in the euthyroid rats: dose-response, time course and demonstration of partial refractoriness to a second dose of thyrotropin-releasing hormone. Endocrinology 102:1775.
Obregon MJ, Pascual A, Mallol J, Morreale de Escobar G, Escobar del Rey F (1980). Evidence against a major role of L-thyroxine at the pituitary level: studies in rats treated with iopanoic acid (Telepaque). Endocrinology 106:1827.
Oppenheimer JH, Schwartz HL, Koerner D, Surks MI (1974). Limited binding capacity sites for L-triiodothyronine in rat liver nuclei, nuclear-cytoplasmatic interrelationships, binding constants and cross-reactivity with L-thyroxine. J Clin Invest 53:768.
Samuels HH, Tsai JS (1974). Thyroid hormone action. Demonstration of similar receptors in isolated nuclei of rat liver and cultured GH_1 cells. J Clin Invest 53:656.
Schwartz HL, Surks MI, Oppenheimer JH (1971). Quantitation of extrathyroidal conversion of L-thyroxine to 3,5,3'-triiodothyronine in the rat. J Clin Invest 50:1124.
Silva JE, Larsen PR (1977). Pituitary nuclear 3,5,3'-triiodothyronine and thyrotropin secretion: an explanation for the effect of thyroxine. Science 198:617.
Silva JE, Silva S (1981). Interrelationship among serum thyroxine, triiodothyronine, reverse triiodothyronine, and thyroid-stimulating hormone in iodine-deficient pregnant women and their offspring: effects of iodine supplementation. J Clin Endocrinol Metab 52:671.

New Concepts in Thyroid Disease, pages 139–153

THE TREATMENT OF THYROID CANCER

Robert D. Leeper M.D.

Nuclear Medicine Service, Memorial Hospital, New York, U.S.A.

For many years cancer of the thyroid has attracted far more attention from clinicians than its numbers would seem to warrant. There are a number of reasons for this interest. For example, the biology of thyroid cancer is almost unique among cancers. Patients with pulmonary metastases from papillary cancer have been followed for 25 years (Cady et al., 1976) and longer (Leeper) with no great change being seen over the period of observation. No other cancer demonstrates this prolonged survival with pulmonary metastases. On the other hand Giant and Spindle cell cancer of the thyroid, which represents only 6%, of all thyroid cancer (Lieberman et al., 1972), is one of the most malignant soft tissue tumors found in man, and survival after diagnosis averages only six months (Rawson and Leeper, 1968). Medullary carcinoma of the thyroid is unique in that approximately one-third of these cancers are heritable. Medullary cancer also secretes a marker hormone (calcitonin). Measurement of this hormone after stimulation with pentagastrin or calcium allow us to make a preoperative diagnosis with nearly 100% accuracy.

Thyroid cancer is also unique in that it is one of the few cancers known where the radioactive form (^{131}I) of a natural metabolite is highly effective in treating many patients with metastatic differentiated cancer (Leeper, 1973). This effectiveness is also the cause of one of the many controversies in the treatment of differentiated thyroid cancer, since some investigators believe it should be used in almost all cases of differentiated cancer (Mazzaferri et al., 1977; De Groot, 1979) and others believe it should be used only in selected cases (Leeper and Shimaoka, 1980; Pochin, 1971). Another source of controversy concerns the extent of surgery which should be done for differentiated cancer. Is total thyroidectomy with its attendant morbidity from hypoparathyroidism and vocal cord paralysis indicated for all differentiated thyroid cancer (Mazzaferri _et al_., 1977; De Groot, 1979) or does lesser local surgery give the same results in terms of survival as suggested by others (Cady _et al_., 1976; Tollefsen _et al_., 1972). In the following discussion these and other problems will be addressed and the author's personal philosophy of treatment will be outlined.

DIAGNOSIS

No discussion of thyroid cancer is complete without a discussion of thyroid nodules. Thyroid cancer is a rather rare tumor. The American Cancer Society estimated that 9900 clinical thyroid cancers would be diagnosed in the U.S. in 1981 (Silverberg, 1981) and that 1050 deaths would occur. Lieberman's data (Lieberman et al., 1972) shows that approximated 5.6% of thyroid cancer is of the anaplastic Giant and Spindle cell variety. Thus about 50% of the deaths are probably due to anaplastic cancer. On the other hand, thyroid nodules are quite common. The Framingham Study (Vander _et al_., 1968) reported an incidence of 4.3% for the thyroid nodules in a screened population (5127 persons aged 30-60) followed for 15 years. These nodules occurred at a rate of 0.1% year. Nine per cent (19/218) of these nodules had been large enough to have warranted surgery at the time of original screening and subsequently another 45 (21%) operations were performed on the original group of persons with thyroid nodules. Thus in 1968 a total of 64 thyroid operations (29% of the original 218 nodules) had been performed. No thyroid cancer was reported. It is obvious from the above figures that most nodular thyroid glands do not in fact contain clinical thyroid cancer.

The preceding discussion where the term clinical thyroid cancer is emphasized is complicated by another problem, that of the so called occult thyroid cancer. These cancers were originally defined as primary papillary cancers which measured $\lesssim$ 1.5 cm in diameter (Hubert _et al_., 1980). Occult cancers, which represented 24.9% of all papillary cancer, were discovered either because of palpable lateral neck node metastases (55/137) or during the course of other operations (82/137). During an average 25.3 year follow-up only 1 patient (.7%) may have died of disease after various conservative operations which included no total thyroidectomies. In another series occult papillary cancer (with or without modal metastases) constituted 28% of 262 consecutive patients who survived after treatment for papillary cancer but none of 70 patients who died from papillary cancer (Tollefsen et al., 1964).

Occult cancer is found at autopsy (Silverberg and Vidone, 1966; Sampson et al., 1974; Mishiyama et al., 1977), and its reported frequency varies according to the methods used in finding it. Mishiyama et al. (1977), sectioned thyroids at two to three mm intervals and examined each slice microscopically and found a 13% incidence. Sampson et al. (1974) made the same size slices and examined only suspicious lesions microscopically. His reported incidence was 5.6% for Olmstead County, Minnesota and 17.9% for unexposed persons in Hiroshima and Nagasaki. It was said that most of these occult cancers occur only in older patients but this is a function of the age at which most people die. A large series with more young deaths included will be required to resolve the question as to whether or not there is an age related increase in the incidence of occult thyroid tumors.

The significance of occult tumors lies not in their lethal potential which must be small but in their contribution to incidence statistics. Cady et al. (1976) states that currently 33% of differentiated cancer is of the occult variety at operations. Tollefsen's et al. (1964) figures indicate that approximately 25% of papillary cancer is occult cancer.

When the search for thyroid cancer becomes more aggressive and more operations are performed more and more occult lesions will be included in the incidence figures. For example, in the report by Favus et al. (1976) on radiation induced thyroid cancer 270 of 1056 patients examined were advised to have operations because of palpable thyroid abnormalities (174) or abnormal thyroid scans showing cold areas (96). Sixty thyroid cancers were found in 182 patients who were actually operated on and who had records available for analysis. Of these cancers only 11 (18%) were of non-occult size. Assuming that the screening procedures detected most of the thyroid cancer in the group, the incidence of thyroid cancer in the screened population was 9.5% a figure within the reported ranges for autopsy proven occult cancer. If the screening procedure did not find the majority of cancers (63% of cancers did not correlate to palpation on scan findings (Favus et al., 1976) then one is faced with the problem of considering prophylactic thyroidectomy in radiated patients if these small lesions are considered to have lethal potential. Because of these and other considerations, we treat findings in the thyroid of adult irradiated patients in the same manner as we treat patients who have no radiation history.

Clinical single nodules have been considered to be an indication for operation in the past but single nodules constituted from 61 to 67% of all nodules in reported studies (Vander et al., 1968; Kendall and Condon, 1969; Sanfelippo et al., 1963). Single nodules constituted 74% of 81 nodular thyroids referred to the Nuclear Medicine Service for thyroid scans in 1975 (Table I). This figure is somewhat higher than in other reported series and is explained by the fact that the physical examination was made while the patient was lying supine under the scanner with the neck hyperextended. Small lesions are difficult to palpate in this position. Nodules less than 1.5 cm represented only 12% of all nodules. Nodules of this size are much less likely to come to the patients notice or to be found on routine physical examinations. However, many of these smaller nodules will be found during screening examinations when nodules are specifically sought for (Vander et al., 1968; Favus et al., 1976).

Scanning procedures have been used to select patients for operation but these too are relatively non specific. The presence of a cold nodule has been reported to be associated with thyroid cancers in from 10% to 20% of cases. These figures are probably high, however, due to the fact that obvious cancers are included in the series. Several studies have shown that 60-70% (Kendall and Condon, 1969; Shimaoka et al., 1969) of all clinical cancer is considered to be suspicious prior to diagnosis because of distant metastasis, lymphadenopathy, rapid growth, vocal cord paralysis, etc. The presence or absence of cold nodules is also a function of the size of the presenting nodule. Table II shows that small nodules whether benign or malignant are much less likely to be cold than larger nodules, depending on the techniques used for scanning.

Sonography has also been used to select patients for thyroidectomy on the basis that cystic lesions are unlikely to be cancerous. However, no more than 25% of surgically removed lesions have been shown to be cystic in whole or in part and the presence of cystic lesions does not eliminate

Table I - Scan findings in 81 Nodular Goiters.

Scan	Classification			Clinical					
	(%)	Single	(%)	(%)	Multiple	(%)	(%)	Total	(%)
Cold	(53)	32	(39)	(38)	8	(10)	(49)	40	(49)
Homogeneous	(33)	20	(25)	(62)	13	(16)	(41)	33	(41)
Hot	(13)	8	(10)		-----		(10)	8	(10)
Total	(100)	60	(74)	(100)	21	(26)	(100)	81	(100)

Results obtained in 81 consecutive patients referred for 99 TcO4- rectilinear scans performed in the Nuclear Medicine Service Memorial Hospital 1975. Clinical classification made while patient was under the scanner.
Percentages to the right in the columns refer to the entire group and those to the left refer to the column only.

Table II - Single Nodules. Effect of Nodule Size on Scan Classification.

	SIZE (cm)			
Scan*	0 - 1.5	1.5 - 3.0	> 3.0	Total
	# (%)	# (%)	# (%)	# (%)
Cold	3 (30)	20 (63)	9 (90)	32 (62)
Homogeneous	7 (70)	12 (37)	1 (10)	20 (38)
Total	10 (100)	32 (100)	10 (100)	52 (100)

* Hot nodules excluded.

the possibility of cancer.

It is probable that needle aspiration and cytologic examination of the aspirate is the single best examination to determine the presence of cancer in a nodule at this time. This procedure is accurate in predicting the presence of a cancer in about 64% of cases and the benign nature of a lesion in 96% of cases (Exelby and Frazell, 1969). In patients with undetermined aspirates (29%) cancer was present in 19%. It is sometimes impossible for a trained pathologist to determine the malignancy of a lesion when an entire surgical specimen is available for examination. Currently, we believe that the best group of examinations which will most accurately predict the presence or absence of malignancy in a nodule are a skillful physical exam, a thyroid scan with $^{99m}TcO_4$ in patients with nodules greater than 2.5 cm in size (for autonomous nodules), fine needle aspiration, and a serum calcitonin determination to rule out the presence of medullary cancer.

TREATMENT

Once the diagnosis of thyroid cancer is established the controversial area of treatment must be approached. As stated previously these controversies arise because of the modest lethality of differentiated thyroid cancers, their unique biologic behavior, and the failure in most reports to accurately stage disease. In a recent report the twenty year gross mortality for papillary cancer was 11%, and for follicular cancer was 24%. These deaths included 3 operative deaths, 3 patients who had small foci of Giant and Spindle cell metaplasia at the time of diagnosis, 26 deaths in patients with inoperable disease or distant metastases, and some deaths from other causes where the patient had thyroid cancer present at the time of death. The maximal 20 year gross death rate for patients with operable differentiated cancer treated by a variety of surgical techniques was 11%. Cady et al. (1976) came to the conclusion that survival did not correlate well with the extent of surgery. In addition, only 1.7% (2/121) of patients aged 50 years of age or less with operable papillary cancer who were placed on thyroid hormone suppression died whereas 13 of 196 (6.6%) patients died who did not receive thyroid hormone replacement. The recurrence rate after surgery was also significantly decreased by thyroid hormone replacement in another study of papillary cancer (Mazzaferri et al., 1977). It appears that thyroid hormone suppression by itself significantly affects survival and the need for total thyroidectomy becomes less apparent. Total thyroidectomy has been advocated (Mazzaferri et al., 1977; De Groot, 1979) because of reports of multifocal disease and in order to prepare the patient for radioiodine therapy. Cady et al. (1976) and Tollefsen et al. (1972) disagree with this approach and believe that the morbidity associated with total thyroidectomy (in the absence of contralateral involvement) is not warranted in view of the benign course exhibited by most differentiated cancer. Total thyroidectomy is not necessary in preparation for ^{131}I therapy since normal thyroid tissue can be ablated with ^{131}I, thus avoiding the surgical risks of total thyroidectomy.

The routine use of radioiodine following surgery for differentiated cancers is also a subject which arouses controversy. Those advocating such treatment do so because of the high rate of multifocality (Mazzaferri _et al._, 1977; De Groot, 1979) in papillary cancer. The advocates suggest that this multifocal disease is eliminated by radiation from nearby normal cells which concentrate ^{131}I. However this has never been shown. Advocates also point to decreased recurrence rates (Mazzaferri _et al._, 1979) as an indication for routine ^{131}I ablation. At our institution only selected patients are given ablative doses of ^{131}I. Our indications for routine ablation of remaining ^{131}I attracting tissue in the thyroid bed are shown in Table III. All patients below the age of 21 receive routine ablation since at least 20% will have distant pulmonary metastases (Harness _et al._, 1971; Cady _et al._, 1979) and many of these metastases are so small as not to be seen on routine chest x-rays. Because no amount of surgery can cure lung metastases, and since so many of these younger patients will have bilateral node disease, we do not advocate extensive surgery in these patients, since ^{131}I will be used in any event.

Ablation in patients ages 21-40 is reserved only for patients with known residual disease after surgery, distant metastases and recurrent disease. Although routine ablation of all patients in this group will prevent some recurrences (Mazzaferri _et al._, 1977) these recurrences are rarely associated with death and can be easily treated with ^{131}I if they occur. Cady _et al._ (1979) has shown that the death rate for operable disease in patients with papillary cancer under the age of 50 and follicular cancer under the age of 40 at diagnosis was only 1% (2/198) in the years 1951-1960 (minimum follow-up 15 years). This was at a time when thyroid hormone suppression was being used on a regular basis and when the selective use of ^{131}I was starting. The possible risks of routine ^{131}I ablation and further therapy if metastatic disease is found became an important consideration at this death rate.

Table III - Indications for ^{131}I thyroid ablation*.

	Pathology	
Age	Papillary	Follicular
0-20	All	All
21-40	Selected	Selected
41-50	Selected	All
51+	Uncertain	All

*See text for explanation and National for indications.

For older patients with follicular cancer we recommend routine thyroid ablation in order to discover distant metastases earlier and treat them before bulk of disease makes successful ^{131}I therapy impossible. At this point, we are not certain as to the correct course to take for papillary cancer diagnosed in patients over the age of 50. This uncertainty stems from our inability to show any beneficial effect of ^{131}I on distant metastases in this age group and our suspicions that radiation in any form may cause some papillary cancer to convert into Giant and Spindle cell cancer (Leeper, 1973).

DOSE SELECTION

The dose selection for thyroid ablation is also a subject of controversy. Some authors (Kuini and Klingensmith, 1980) have reported that 30 mCi ^{131}I will successfully ablate normal thyroid tissue in a significant proportion of patients whereas other authors have stated the opposite (Benua et al., 1962). This is important for two reasons. If routine ablation is practiced then it is advisable to keep the dose of ^{131}I as low as possible since each mCi of ^{131}I gives from 1/3-2/3 rads to blood (De Groot, 1979). Secondly, patients must be hospitalized (in the U.S.) if more than 30 mCi ^{131}I is retained in a patient and this drives the cost of ablation up by several hundred dollars. Currently, we continue to use 75 mCi of ^{131}I as a standard dose for ablation. A single 75 mCi dose successfully ablates thyroid function in 83% of patients (Leeper and Shimaoka, 1980). The morbidity caused by ablative doses of ^{131}I is small and consists primarily of asymtomatic thyroiditis which is easily controlled, even when ablating an entire gland.

Dose selection for therapy is also controversial. Almost all institutions in the United States use an arbitrary dose selection method whereby a standard dose of ^{131}I (upper limit 200 mCi) is given to all patients without regard for the rad dose of blood (De Groot, 1979). Doses are arbitrarily decreased for children or for patients with wide spread pulmonary metastases. If there is minimal metastatic disease present this dose selection method is probably adequate for adults. Some authors suggest retreatment at three to four month intervals (De Groot, 1979) while others (Leeper and Shimaoka, 1980) treat only at yearly intervals. Our policy is the latter because it is our impression that more frequent treatment is associated with an increased frequency of leukemia (Pochin, 1971) probably related to failure to allow maximum bone marrow recovery. No case of leukemia secondary to ^{131}I therapy has been seen at this institution since 1960 in spite of the larger rad doses to blood which we give.

The authors prefers to use a dosimetry procedure using a one mCi ^{131}I tracer dose as described previously (Leeper, 1973; Leeper and Shimaoka, 1979). Briefly, the procedure entails the drawing of blood at 4 hours and daily for four days after the oral administration of one mCi ^{131}I and counting radio activity (expressed as % dose/l) in an aliquot of blood. Counting rates are compared to a standard made up simultaneously with the tracer dose. By integration under the resulting curve the β rad dose to blood (the critical organ) can be calculated (assuming 10 rads/liter/mCi day). The dose to blood after the four days is calculated using physical decay only. Twenty four hour urines are also collected, volumes measured, urine samples counted, and the % retention in the body determined over the study period. From this determination, a γ contribution to whole body radiation can be calculated by integration under the retention curve. The gamma contribution can be calculated by the formula rads = 20.4 rads/mCi day/kg x 0.4 where 0.4 is the fraction of γ radiation affecting blood. Gamma and β contributions are summed and the rad dose to blood/mCi can be estimated for each patient. Doses of ^{131}I are calculated to deliver 200 rads to blood (the usual limiting dose), no more than 120 mCi retained at 48 hours, or no more than 80 mCi retained at 48 hours in the presence of diffuse lung metastases. Using these criteria, we have observed no leukemia, permanent bone marrow suppression, or pulmonary fibrosis. The only fatality clearly related to ^{131}I occurred in an elderly female with long neglected follicular cancer metastatic to the lungs. After the usual preparation this patient received 294 mCi ^{131}I. Within 24 hours the patient developed a tumor necrosis syndrome (rapidly rising serum potassium, urea nitrogen, uric acid and phosphorus). Severe hemoptysis occurred and the patient died within a few days. The patients death was clearly due to rapid necrosis of large amounts of tumor.

This dosimetry procedure has allowed us to give an average single dose of ^{131}I of 309 mCi with a range of 70 to 654 mCi. These data were obtained from 120 doses given to 70 patients with metastatic differentiated cancer seen since 1973. Eight children (16 years of age or less) have received single doses of ^{131}I ranging from 128 mCi to 494 mCi without discernible permanent depression or pulmonary fibrosis. Thirty patients received more than one dose of ^{131}I. Of these 6 had a cumulative dose of over 1000 mCi.

One patient received 2.163 curies of ^{131}I given in 6 doses over 6 years prior to death. Three patients received an estimated 1000 rads or more to blood given over five to six years. At these high dose levels, the bone marrow is chronically but not completely suppressed and further treatment is usually not possible. In those patients given more than one therapeutic dose of ^{131}I the size of subsequent doses becomes a gross indicator of the future success or failure to treatments.

Of seven patients who died of differentiated cancer and no other cause only one patient had received a calculated higher dose ($>$10%) than the previous dose prior to death whereas 6 of 8 patients who were cured (by physical findings, x-ray evidence, and scans) received doses of ^{131}I 10% or more higher than the previous dose ($p < .02$). This effect is shown in Table IV. Rising dose sizes indicate decreased tumor burden and therefore, less ^{131}I retention in the body.

The results of treatment have been reported previously (Leeper, 1973) and results obtained in the last 70 patients treated are shown in Table V. Twenty-one patients died du-

Table IV - Inverse Correlation between Tumor Burden and Dose Size*

Date	Calculated Therapy Dose (mCi)	Neck Uptake % (In tumor) at 24 Hours.
2/8/75	75 (Ablation)	
5/1/75	70	43
7/1/75	88	35
4/16/76	169	--
4/14/77	213	26
4/25/78	271	--
4/18/79	640	0.6

* Patient ST had massive bilateral cervical lymphadenopathy and pulmonary metastases. There was no evidence of disease by radiographic studies, scans, or physical examination in 1980.

ring the 8 year period (1974 through 1981) all with metastatic disease present. Of these patients one died after surgery at another institution, one died immediately after a calcium infusion given because of a modestly elevated calcitonin level, one died of a cerebro-vascular accident following anticoagulant therapy for thrombophlebitis, and one died as the result of a second primary lung carcinoma. Of those who died of thyroid cancer and no other cause, one died of anaplastic conversion of an original papillary cancer after two ^{131}I treatments and the tumor necrosis death has already been mentioned. Of the 17 deaths related to thyroid cancer (including the tumor necrosis death) five were under the age of 40 and 12 (91%) were older than 40 at the age of diagnosis. In some cases there was a prolonged treatment delay in the younger patients.

Twenty-one patients were "cured". Only four (19%) were older than 40 years of age at diagnosis and 5 (24%) were younger than age 16 at diagnosis though not necessarily at the time of ^{131}I treatment. Thirteen of the 21 "cured" patients had no evidence of disease after a single treatment,

Table V - Status of 70 Patients with Metastatic differentiated thyroid cancer treated with ^{131}I 1974-1981.

Status	N=	Number of Treatments*						Total mCi (Ave)
		1	2	3	4	5	6	
Cured	21	13	6	1	0	0	1	9715(463)
Dead of Disease	17	9	3	3	0	1	1	10715(630)
Dead of Other Causes	4	2	2	0	0	0	0	2271(568)
Under Treatment	19	10	6	1	2	0	0	9765(514)
Living with Disease No further Rx	6	5	1	0	0	0	0	2795(466)
Lost to followup	3	2	1					1136(379)
Total	70	41	19	5	2	1	2	36397(520)

* Each treatment calculated to give approximately 200 rads to blood in most cases. Treatment given at yearly intervals.

6 required 2 treatments, one required 3 treatments and one had 6 treatments. Cumulative doses ranged from 183 mCi to 1131 mCi (excluding ablation doses).

The initial dose of ^{131}I was less than 200 mCi in 13 (19%) of the seventy and greater in 57 or 81%. Six patients received less than 150 mCi. If a standard 200 mCi dose had been given to all patients 19% would have received more than 200 rads to blood and might have been subjected to a risk of permanent bone marrow suppression. Of perhaps more importance, is the fact that 81% of patients would have received less than an optimal amount of ^{131}I. If 150 mCi doses had been routinely given to the patient described in Table IV, 7 or 8 treatments would have been necessary, some of which might have given 400 rads or more to blood.

The major morbidity from these doses of ^{131}I is parotitis and permanent parotid failure which may eventually result in poor dentition. Currently, we are investigating methods to prevent this complication.

CONCLUSION

Various controversies relating to the treatment of thyroid cancer have been presented and our own philosophy outlined. Currently, we feel that only those thyroid nodules found to have suspicious findings on fine needle aspiration should be surgically removed, whether or not there is a history of radiation. Total thyroidectomy should be performed in patients with papillary or follicular cancer only in those patients who have bilateral disease at the time of surgery. Routine ^{131}I ablation and therapy if required should be performed in all patients under the age of 20, in patients with recurrent, unresectable or metastatic disease in patients ages 21 to 40 years of age, and in all patients over the age of 40 with follicular cancer. In our judgement, dosimetry should be performed in all patients who are to be given ^{131}I therapy for metastatic disease in order to optimize doses safely.

REFERENCES

Benua RS, Cicale NR, Sonenberg M, et al.(1962) The relation of radioiodine dosimetry to results and complications in the treatment of metastatic thyroid cancer. Am. J. Roentgenol. and Rad. Therapy 87: 171.

Cady B, Sedwick CE, Meissner WA, Bookwalter JR, Romagosa V, Werber J (1976) Changing clinical, pathologic, therapeutic and survival patterns in differentiated thyroid carcinoma. Ann. of Surg. 183: 541.

Cady B, Sedwick CE, Meissner WA, et al. (1979) Risk factor analysis in differentiated thyroid cancer. Cancer 43: 810.

De Groot L (1979) Thyroid Neoplasia. In Endocrinology (De Groot Ed.) Grune and Stratton, New York, pp 509-521.

Exelby PG, Frazell EL (1969) Carcinoma of the thyroid in children. Surg. Clin.N.A. 49: 249.

Favus MJ, Schneider AB, Stachura ME, et al. (1976) Thyroid cancer appearing as a late consequence of head-and-neck irradiation: Evaluation of 1056 patients. N. Engl. J. Med. 294: 1019.

Harness JK, Thompson NW, Nishiyama RN (1971) Childhood thyroid carcinoma. Arch. Surg. 102: 278.

Hubert JP, Kiernan PD, Beahrs OH, McConahey WM, Woolner LB (1980) Occult papillary carcinoma of the thyroid. Arch. Surg. 115: 394.

Kuini CC, Klingensmith WC (1980) Failure of low doses of ^{131}I to ablate residual thyroid tissue following surgery

for thyroid cancer. Radiology 137: 773.
Kendall LW, Condon RE (1969) Prediction of malignancy in solitary thyroid nodules. Lancet 1: 1071.
Leeper RD. Unpublished observations.
Leeper RD (1973) The effect of ^{131}I therapy on survival of patients with metastatic papillary or follicular thyroid carcinoma. JCEM 36: 1143.
Leeper RD, Shimaoka K (1980) Treatment of metastatic thyroid cancer. Clin. Endo. Metab. 9: 383.
Lieberman PH, Foote FW, Schottenfeld D (1972) A study of the pathology of thyroid cancer, 1930-1960. MSKCC Cancer Bulletin 2: 7.
Mazzaferri EL, Young RL, Oertel JE, Kemmerer WT, Page CP (1977) Papillary carcinoma: the impact of therapy in 576 patients. Medicine (Baltimore) 56: 171.
McGowen KD, Adler RA, Nasser G, et al. (1976) Low dose radioiodine ablation in post surgical patients with thyroid cancer. Am. J. Med. 61: 52.
Mishiyama RH, Ludwig GK, Thompson NW (1977) The prevalence of small papillary thyroid carcinomas in 100 consecutive necropsies in an American Population. In Radiation Associated Thyroid Carcinoma (Ed) De Groot, LG, Grune and Stratton, New York, pp 123-135.
Pochin EE (1971) Radioiodine Therapy. In The Thyroid (Ed.) Werner SE, Ingbar SH, Harper and Row, New York, pp 467-475.
Rawson RW, Leeper RD (1968) Factors influencing benignancy versus malignancy of thyroid neoplasms. In Thyroid Neoplasia (Ed.) Young S, Inman DR, Academic Press, New York, pp 159.
Silverberg E (1981) Cancer Statistics 1981. CA-A Cancer Journal for Physicians 31: 13.
Silverberg SG, Vidone RA (1966) Carcinoma of the thyroid in surgical and postmortem material. Ann. Surg. 164: 291.
Sampson RJ, Woolner LB, Bahn RC, et al. (1974) Occult thyroid carcinoma in Olmsted County, Minnesota: Prevalence at autopsy compared with that in Hiroshima and Nagasaki, Japan. Cancer 34: 2072.
Sanfelippo PM, Bearhs OH, McConahey WM, et al. (1973) Indications for thyroidectomy. Mayo Clinic Proc. 48: 269.
Shimaoka K, Badillo J, Sokal JE, et al. (1962) Clinical differentiation between thyroid cancer and benign goiter. JAMA 181: 179.
Tollefsen H, Shah JP, Huvos AG (1972) Papillary carcinoma of the thyroid. Recurrence in the thyroid gland after initial surgical treatment. Am. J. Surg. 124: 468.

Tollefsen HR, DeCosse JJ, Hutter RVP (1964) Papillary carcinoma of the thyroid. A clinical and pathological study of 70 fatal cases. Cancer 17: 1035.
Vander JB, Gaston EA, Dawber TR (1968) The significance of nontoxic thyroid nodules: Final report of a 15 year study on the incidence of thyroid malignancy. Ann Internal. Medicine 69: 537.

New Concepts in Thyroid Disease, pages 155–167

UNUSUAL MANIFESTATIONS OF THYROTOXICOSIS

Geraldo Medeiros-Neto

Thyroid Laboratory,Hospital Das Clínicas,Faculdade de Medicina da Universidade de São Paulo
São Paulo,Brazil

Thyroxicosis is most often caused by the uncontrolled synthesis of hormones in toxic nodular goiter and by the diffuse thyroid hyperplasia of Graves' disease.JT also arises from thyrotropin-secreting pituitary tumors and from thyroid-stimulating substances (HCG =human chorionic gonadotropin) secreted by hydatiform moles,choriocarcinomas and seminomas. It may also be induced by the release of thyroid hormones during an episode of subacute thyroiditis or radiation injury to the gland or by uncontrolled release of T_3 and T_4 from metastatic thyroid carcinoma.Thyrotoxicosis factitia is a syndrome in which the patient may chronically ingest an excess of thyroid hormone in an attempt to lose weight or, most common in our experience,is the patient who is inadvertedly rendered hyperthyroid by a physician in an attempt to correct a laboratory result such as a low serum T_4 concentration due to a previous therapeutic trial with T_3.Thyrotroxicosis factitia may also be present when a physician wishes to supress thyrotropin secretion from the pituitary using increasing large doses of a combined tablet containing both T_4 and T_3 in instances of thyroid carcinoma (post-operatively).On the other hand special terms have been used in the literature to describe certain variations of the fundamental picture of thyrotoxicosis.Thus,apathetic hyperthyroidism is used to describe certain cases,usually among older patients in whom the symptoms are mild or veiled, although the serum concentration of thyroid hormones is relatively high.Another term frequently used is masked hyperthyroidism implying that the symptoms produced by an actual state of hyperthyroidism ,more closely resemble another disorder,chiefly heart disease and its manifestations.

Apart from Graves' disease and toxic adenoma, hyperthyroidism may occur in rarer syndromes such as:

1. Metastatic thyroid carcinoma.

Thyroid cancer probably produces hyperthyroidism when the mass of metastatic tissue, of low hormone producing capacity, is sufficiently big to provide an excess of thyroid hormones. The syndrome was first reported by Leiter et al (1946) and since then, 17 new patients were reported in the literature. In one patient reported by Bloise et al (1963) the size of the osseous metastasis was big enough to account for a very large hormonal production (PBI : 18.4 ug/dl) and progressively lead the patient to a thyrotoxic crisis and electrolyte disturbances. More recently Sung and Cavalieri (1973) reported on T_3 thyrotoxicosis due to metastatic thyroid carcinoma. This finding was confirmed by Mornex et al (1976) who reported on a patient who developed bone and liver metastasis 9 years after surgical ablation of a differentiated carcinoma of thyroid. Suprisingly the patient had a clear increase of serum T_3 but only a minor elevation of serum T_4 (Table 1), and the TSH secretion was blocked.

Table 1: LABORATORY FINDINGS IN HYPERTHYROIDISM CAUSED BY ACTIVE THYROID CANCER METASTASES

Patient	Age years	Metastases	PBI ug/dl	T_4 ug/dl	T_3 ng/dl	Reference
(F)	56	Bone-Lung	18.4	-	-	Bloise et al (1968)
(M)	52	Bone	-	4.2	820	Sung et al (1973)
(F)	66	Bone-Liver	13.3	12.3	440	Mornex et al (1976)
(F)	64	Bone	8.9	6.2	536	Medeiros-Neto et al (1971)

Exogenous TSH increased iodine uptake in the thyroid but not in the metastasis. We have also reported (Medeiros-Neto 1971) a patient with a large bone metastasis and a clinical picture of thyrotoxicosis with abnormally high serum T_3 concentration and normal serum T_4 level (Figure 1). It may be possible that the malignant metastatic tissue is relatively deprived of iodide and presents structural and functional heterogenity at follicular level that would favour a preferential secretion of T_3 such as observed in endemic goiter.

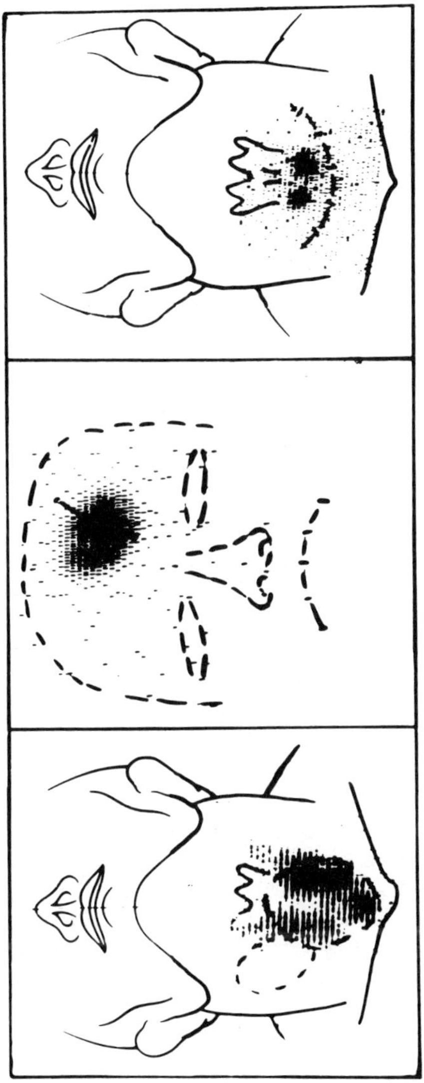

Fig.1- A 64 year-old female with metastatic follicular carcinoma of the thyroid gland to the frontal bone and clinical signs of thyrotoxicosis. Serum T_4 was 6.2ug/dl but serum T_3 was 536 ng/dl (T_3 toxicosis).A large amount of an abnormal serum iodoprotein was detected by column chromatography (Medeiros-Neto 1971)

2.Inappropriate secretion of thyroid-stimulating hormone (TSH)

In the conventional forms of thyrotoxicosos,i.e.,Graves' disease or toxic adenoma,serum TSH is suppressed so that TSH is undetectable in serum and does not increase after the administration of TRH,in the presence of elevated total and free serum thyroid hormones.Thus patients in whom free serum thyroid hormones are elevated but in whom TSH is detectable are considered to have inappropiate TSH secretion even if the level of TSH falls within the usual "normal range".These patients may be thyrotoxic or euthyroid and they may harbor pituitary tumors.In Table 2 we have classified these patients in two major groups, without a pituitary tumor and those with a radiologic and laboratory evidence for a pituitary adenoma:

Table 2:HYPERSECRETION OF TSH ASSOCIATED WITH THYROTOXICOSIS

I.Selective pituitary resistance to elevated serum T_4 and T_3 levels

II.Pituitary tumors

Acromegaly,Galactorrhea-Amenorrhea
Elevated GH or PRL in some patients
No further increase in TSH after TRH
No suppression of serum TSH after T_4
Tsh is suppressed by glucocorticoids and SRF
Hypersecretion of alpha-subunits/TSH
Absence of Thyroid-binding Immunoglobulins (TSAb)

Again,this classification is dependent on whether hypersecretion of TSH is associated with a pituitary tumor (type II) or not (type I).In the latter group patients who are resistant to the action of thyroid hormones (Refetoff syndrome),and,who therefore require elevated circulating levels of both T_4 and T_3 to maintain eumetabolic state are not included.Other patients are resistant selectively or predominantly at pituitary level such as one patient described by Gershengorn & Weintraub (1975).In this young woman TSH induced hyperthyroidism was caused by a selective pituitary resistance to the blocking action of thyroid hormone.This young patient(9 years old)received various series of treatment with PTU for hyperthyroidism and was finally thyroidectomized at age 13.Histologic examination revealed diffuse parenchymatous hyperplasia.At the age of 18 she was again hyperthyroid(T_4=12.7ug/dl,T_3 220ng/dl) and TSH was not only absolutely elevated (9.3uU/ml)but was inappropriate relative to the elevated thyroid hormones levels normally associated with suppressed TSH.Stimulation by TRH resulted in a rise in serum levels of TSH to 62uU/ml and serum T_3 rose to 420 ng/dl (180 min).Thus TSH response was twice normal and similar to that usually found in primary hypothyroidism. The rise in T_3 indicated that the measured TSH was biologically effective.Although the patient' s TSH response to TRH was partially blunted by exogenous T_3 administration there was still a marked response to 23 uU/ml.The etiology of this patient' s hyperthyroidism was TSH hypersecretion due to a selective resistance of the thyrotroph to the action of the thyroid hormones.

The results of four other patients of this group have been published and the general picture of this syndrome may be summarized as follows(Mornex 1981)

1.Onset of hyperthyroidism was very precocious(7-14 years old)
2.Duration of thyrotoxicosis was very long (23 years)
3.Goiter is usually large and has been surgically removed previous to the demonstration of TSH hypersecretion
4.Hyperthyroidism is usually clinically mild
5.TSH is elevated and stimulated by TRH
6.In all cases the elevated TSH was suppressed by exogenous T_3 and dexamethasone
7.Alpha subunits is usually normal.

Pituitary tumors associated with hypersecretion of TSH and hyperthyroidism have been described (Mornex,1981-Hamon, 1981).In the 21 cases so far published only 9 fulfilled all the criteria for a diagnosis of hyperthyroidism secondary to a pituitary thyreotrophic adenoma.In 12 cases the complete picture was not present but the presumption is sufficient to draw the general features of htis disease:

1.Age between 40-58 years old and goiter is present in the mayority of the patients.
2.TSH levels above 10 uU/ml despite high levels of T_4 and T_3.
3.TRH failed to further increase TSH above basal level.
4.TSH was not suppressible with exogenous T_3.
5.The pituitary adenoma is commonly associated with other hormonal disturbances (acromegaly,Galactorrhea-Amenorrhea,hypopituitarism).
6.Clear increase of alpha subunits with normal TSH level; the alpha subunit was not stimulated (TRH) or suppressible (T_3).

Measurement of the individual alpha and beta subunits

of TSH has been useful in differentating those patients with TSH-induced hyperthyroidism who have a pituitary tumor from those without a tumor(Kourides,I,1980).The patients with a pituitary tumor have had markedly elevated serum alpha subunits levels relative to their TSH level but undetectable beta subunits of TSH:

Table 3:TSH AND ALPHA SUBUNIT CONCENTRATIONS IN PATIENTS WITH TSH-INDUCED HYPERTHYROIDISM(KOURIDES,1980)

	TSH uU/ml	ALPHA SUBUNIT ng/ml
Pituitary tumor (n = 7)	1.7 - 8.8	12.5 - 105.0
No pituitary tumor	9.3 - 160	0.5 - 5.2

The non-tumor patientes showed modestly increased serum concentration of both alpha and beta subunits of TSH but predominantly increased TSH secretion.Pituitary tumor patients demonstrated non-significant increase in the concentration of TSH or its subunits after TRS administration, while the patients without a pituitary tumor showed both increased TSH and subunit secretion.

Azukizawa et al (1980) recently described a 28 year old woman with overt hyperthyroidism and an enlarged sella turcica.Her serum TSH levels were elevated in association with high serum concentrations of both T_4 and T_3 and TSH was not responsive to TRH stimulation or exogenous T_3 suppression.Corticosteroid administration,however,markedly decreased serum TSH concentration and flattened the diurnal variation of serum TSH.The pituitary tumor was identified as a TSH secreting chromophobe adenoma.Subsequently the patient developed a clinical and laboratory picture of Graves' disease with mild exophthalmos,positive MHT test and high levels of TSAb stimulating antibodies.These results indicate that hyperthyroidism initially attributable to a TSH-secreting pituitary adenoma,later,on the course of the disease,was caused by a typical Graves' disease.

Recently we had the opprotunity of examining a patient with a pituitary TSH secreting tumor in the "Hospital Clínico de la Universidad Católica" in Santiago de Chile.This patient studied by Dr.Lopez and Rodriguez developed hyperthyroidism in April 1978 (T_4 =12.8 ug/dl,T_3 =550 ng/dl) but the serum TSH was abnormally high (12.0-29.0uU/ml)and not stimulated by TRH but suppressed to normal levels (2.5uU/ml) after dexamethasone.One year later(1978) he was operated for a pituitary adenoma and remained euthyroid until 1979, when,again,presented clinical and laboratory evidence of thyrotoxicosis (T_4 = 13.1 ug/dl,T_3 =650ng/ml) and a normal serum TSH concentration (1.2-2.4 uU/ml).He was started on PTU (400mg/day) followed by 16mCi of ^{131}I and remained euthyroid up to the present examination (August 1981).Presumably the patient developed a clinical picture of Graves' disease after the thyrotoxicosis produced by the inappropriate TSH secretion but this was not confirmed with a positive TSAb test.This case report is similar to the patient reported by Azukizawa et al (1980)and indicates the possibility of dual ethiology(not concomitant) for thyrotoxicosis.

3.Trophoblastic disease and hyperthyroidism

Biochemical thyroid hyperactivity in patients with trophoblastic disease is due to the presence of an abnormal thyroid stimulator,not related to immunoglobulins.HCG has the same molecular weight as TSH and cross-reacts with TSH antibodies.Most patients are clinically euthyroid but there have been reported some with clinical hyperthyroidism. Hyperthyroidism with a circulating TSH-like substance has also been seen in a patient with a testicular embryonal carcinoma(Streghigel,N.,1964).Recently Chan et al (1980) reported on thyroid function of 20 patients with molar pregnancy and 10 with choriocarcinoma.All patients were clinically euthyroid and showed normal thyroid hormones, TSH,alpha and TSH-beta subunits as well as beta-HCG were measured by RIA fortnightly,before and during treatment. Seven out of eight patients had a blunted TSH response to TRH and,after remission,all gave a positive TSH response to TRH.Abnormal immunoglobulins (TSAb) stimulating the thyroid gland were not found in these patients.Results of the serum thyroid hormones are shown in Table 4.

In brief these patients have markedly elevated serum T_3 levels,usually accompained by T_4 and FTI in the upper normal limit(T_3 thyrotoxicosis).Alpha subunit concentration paralleled that of HCG and it is likely that the thyroid stimulator in molar tissue has the same alpha subunit as

HCG and TSH.Furthermore the demonstration of normal TSH-beta levels before and after treatment and that HCG and TSH-competing activities found in the molar extracts strongly suggests that the abnormal thyroid stimulator may be HCG.

Table 4:FREE THYROXINE INDEX (FTI)AND SERUM T_3 IN TROPHOBLASTIC DISEASE
(Chan et al,1980)

Patient group (n)*	FTI	T_3 (nmol/L)
Molar Pregnancy (9)	165 $\pm$ 32.7	4.6 $\pm$ 1.0
Choriocarcinoma (10)	190 $\pm$ 32.2	6.1 $\pm$ 1.3
Normal range	52-154	1.08-2.76

* All patients had a negative TSH response to TRH,TSAb test was also NEGATIVE

4.Lymphocytic thyroiditis with spontaneously resolving hyperthyroidism

Lymphocytic thyroiditis with spontaneously resolving hyperthyroidism (LT - SRT) is a new form of thyrotoxicosis that has been recognized with an increasing frequency in the past decade (Nikolai,1979).It is usually manifested as a mild degree of thyroid hyperfunction with a non tender enlarged thyroid gland,elevated serum concentrations of both T_4 and T_3,a depressed thyroid iodine uptake and spontaneous resolution in 2 to 6 months(Figure 2).The sedimentation rate is normal in 50% of the patients or slightly elevated (up to 50mm/hr)in contrast with subacute thyroiditis in which the sedimentation rate is almost always higher than 50mm/hs.There is no response to TRH as in other forms of hyperthyroidism.Also the thyroid does not respond to exogenous TSH stimulation,indicating a damaged thyroid rather than merely thyroid suppression due to elevated T_4 and T_3 levels.Needle biposy of the thyroid has shown a focal or diffuse lymphocytic thyroiditis.It is quite difficult to diagnose LT -SRT from fractitious thyrotoxicosis. A non palpable thyroid should be found on examination of the latter due to thyroid suppression and the gland should respond with an increase in thyroid uptake of RAI after exogenous TSH stimulation.

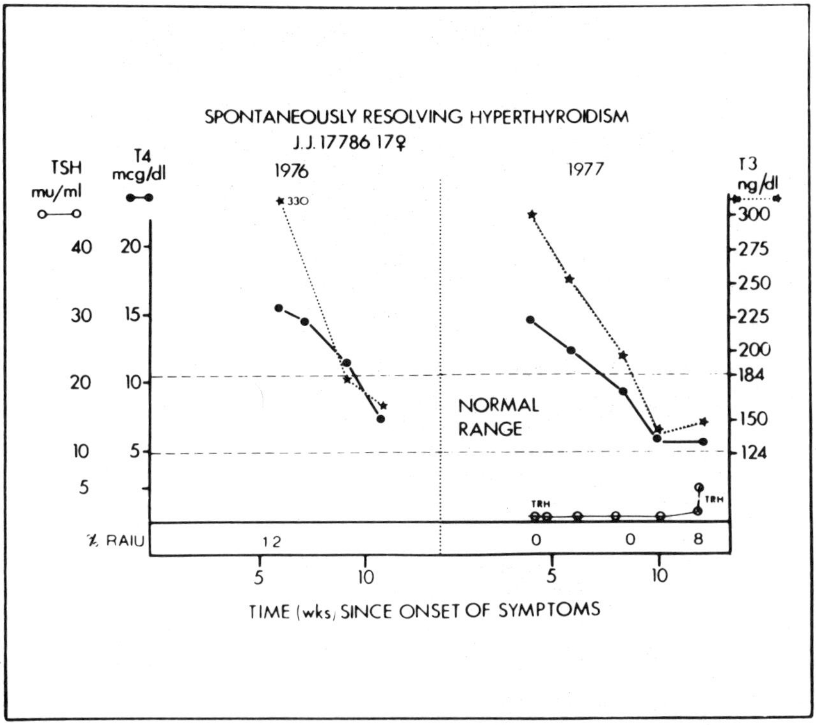

Fig.2-Lymphocytic thyroiditis with spontaneous-resolving thyrotoxicosis.Note the high serum levels of both T_4 and T_3,the blunted TSH response to TRH and the absence of thyroidal uptake of radioiodine (% RAIU).In two occasions there was a spontaneous remission in five weeks(NIKOLAI, 1979).

5.T_3-thyrotoxicosis

Laboratory confirmation of hyperthyroidism most commonly rests on the finding of raised serum levels of thyrotoxine (total and free T_4).Hyperthyroid patients have been described,in whom hypermetabolism can only be abscribed to elevated serum T_3 but normal serum T_4(T_3-thyrotoxicosis).It was first described in 1968 by Hollander and,subsequently,considered that 4% of all patients presenting hyperthyroidism for the first time have T_3

thyrotoxicosis.It may be seen at any phase of Graves' disease but it is more common early in its course and during or following treatment of hyperthyroidism with antithyroid drugs,radioiodine,or surgery.It was also reported in patients with nodular goiter receiving iodinated contrast media (Medeiros-Neto,1977) and in thyrotoxicosis associated with thyroid cancer functionig metastases.

In Chile,an area of relative iodine deficiency,12.5% of hyperthyroid patients had T_3 toxicosis(Hollander,C.S.,1972). All patients (n=12) had diffusely enlarged thyroid glands and thyroid uptake or radioiodine was raised in 8 of them. In 5 patients RAIU was not suppressible with exogenous T_3 administration.Serum T_4 (total and free T_4)levels were normal and serum T_3 levels were raised in all cases(range 360-840ng/dl)

TABLE 5:CLINICAL AND LABORATORY FINDINGS IN T_3 THYROTOXICOSIS (Endemic area,Chile)*

Patients n=12	Age (years	RAI UPTAKE (%)	Serum T_4 Total ug/dl	Serum T_4 Free ng/dl	Serum T_3 ng/dl
9F/3M	23-50	22 - 80 45(n=11)	5.2 to 8.8	1.1 to 1.8	360 - 840
Normal range:		15 - 50	5-11	1.0-2.1	100 - 180

*Hollander,Stevenson,Pineda et al (1972)

A relative preferential and hypersecretion of T_3 may represent an important homeostatic mechanism in the face of inadequate iodide substrate.Therefore the thyroid gland of these patients preferntially secrete more T_3 than T_4 where an adequate iodine intake is present.Heterogeneity within the thyroid gland on a follicular level could also lead to relative iodine deficiency in the smaller,more active follicles which may produce the bulk of the thyroid hormone. Autonomous areas(nodular) could also be the cause of the hypersecretion of T_3 and this syndrome may progress spontaneously to conventional hyperthyroidism with raised levels of both T_3 and T_4 as seen in the goitrous patients who recently arrived to a urban area,previously mentioned.

Abstract

Thyrotoxicosis is a condition characterized by a distorted and accelerated metabolism in most tissues of the body,produced by the action of excess thyroid hormones.More often is caused by toxic adenoma and by the diffuse hyperplasia of Graves-Basedow disease.Nevertheless thyrotoxicosis may arise from active metastases of differentiated thyroid carcinoma .In this case,a high secretion of T_3 (400-890ng/dl) in the presence of normal or bordeline serum T_4(6.8-10.9 ug/dl)was usually observed.Inappropriate secretion of TSH may induce hyperthyroidism either by selective resistance of the pituitary thyrotroph to the action of thyroid hormones or hypersecretion of TSH associated with a pituitary tumor.In the former,TSH was not absolutely elevated (9.3uU/ml)in the presence of high serum T_4 (12.7uU/dl)and T_3(220ng/dl)but TSH response to TRH was twice normal(peak: 62uU/ml)and only suppressed by high dosis of exogenous T_4. Most patients with immunoactive elevated TSH and hyperthyroidism have been shown to have a pituitary tumor associated or not with acromegaly and/or the galactorrhea-amenorrhea syndrome.TSH secreting pituitary tumors consistently demonstrate greater hypersecretion of the free alpha subunit relative to TSH whereas hyperthyroid patients with inappropriate TSH secretion without tumor have normal serum alpha concentration.Thyrotoxicosis or elevated serum thyroid hormones concentration can be readily demonstrated in patients with hydatiform moles or choriocarcinomas and the thyroid stimulating substance has been identified with human chorionic gonadotrofin. T_3-thyrotoxicosis has also been shown to occur frequently in endemic goiter patients with diffuse or multinodular goiter once they are exposed to a higher daily intake of iodine when moving to a urban iodine-rich area or when receiving iodinated contrast media.Exogenous use of thyroid hormones can also trigger hyperthyroidism in a predisposed patient or in an individual with a multinodular goiter.Lymphocytic thyroiditis with a spontaneous-resolving hyperthyroidism is a new form of thyrotoxicosis characterized by elevated serum of both T_4 and T_3,a depressed thyroid iodine uptake and spontaneous resolution in 2-6 months. The thyroid gland is not responsive to exogenous TSH administration and the sedimentation rate is usually below 50mm/hr.Needle biopsy of the thyroid shows a focal or diffuse lymphocytic thyroiditis.

REFERENCES

Azukizawa,M.,Morimoto,S.,Miyai,K.,Miki,T.,Yaby,Y.,Amino,N. Kuma,K.,&Kumahara,Y. 1980 TSH-producing pituitary adenoma associated with Graves' disease in:Thyroid Research VIII, Australian Academy of Sciences,Canberra,p.645

Bloise,W.,Nicolau,W.,Wajchenberg,B.L.,Pieroni,R.R.,Toledo, A.C.,Cintra,A.B.U. 1963 Thyrotoxic crisis and electrlytic disturbances in a patient with functioning metastatic carcinoma of the thyroid J Clin Endocrinol Metab 23:1096

Chan,V.,Wang,C.,Ho,P.C.,Yeung,R.T.T. & Ma,H.K. 1980 Biochemical thyroid hyperfunction in trophoblastic disease in :Stockigt,J.R. and Nagataki,S."Thyroid Research VIII" Austr Acad Sc,Canberra,p.598

Hamon,P.,Baulieu,J.L.,Doumith,R.,Jambart,S.,Turpin,G. 1981 Secretion inappropiée de thyreostimuline N.Presse Med 10:2285

Hersham,J.M.&Higgins,H.P. 1971 Hydatiform mole:a cause of clinical hyperthyroidism New Engl J Med 284:573

Hollander,C.S.,Stevenson,C.Mitisuma,T.,Pineda,C.,Shenkman,L., & Silva,J.E. 1972 T_3 Toxicosis in an Iodine-deficient area Lancet II:1276

Jailer,J.N.,Holub,D.A. 1960 Remission of Graves disease following radiotherapy of a pituitary neoplasm Ann J Med 49:497

Kourides,I.A.,Ridgway,E.C.,Weintraub,B.D.,Bigos,S.T. Gershengorn,M.C.&Maloof,F. 1977 Thyrotropin induced hyper-thyroidism:use of alpha and beta subunit levels to identify patients with pituitary tumours.J Clin Endocrinol Metab 45:534

Kourides,I.A. 1980 Pituitary thyrotropin secretion in thyroid disorders Thyroid Today 3:1-5

Leiter,L.,Seidlm,S.M.,Marinelli,L.D. 1946 Adenocarcinoma of the thyroid with hyperthyroidism and functional metastases.J Clin Endocrinol Metab 6:247

Linquette,M.,Herlant,M.,Fossati,P.,May,J.P.,Decolux,M.& Fourlinnie,J.C. 1969 Adenoma hypophysaire a cellules thyreotropes avec hyperthyroidie Ann Endocrinol (Paris) 30:731

Mornex,R.,Pousset,G.,Briere,J.,Daumont,M. & Paffoy,J.C. 1976 Hypertiroide par metastases autonomes et extintives d' un cancer thyroiden Ann d' Endocrinol (Paris) 37:1113

Medeiros-Neto,G.A.,Ferraz,A.R.,Thom,A.,Serson,D.& Toledo,A.C. 1971 Adenocarcinoma folicular de tireoide com metástases osseas funcionantes.Rev Hosp Clin Fac Med S Paulo 26:233

Mornex,R. 1981 Primary hypersecretion of TSH and its

subunits in TSH induced hyperthyroiidsm 11th European Thyr Association Meeting p.30-36

Mornex,R.,Tommasi,M.,Cure,M,Farcot,J.,Argiazzi,J.&Rousset, b. Hyperthyroide associé ā un hypoituitarisme au cours de l' évolution d' une tumeur sécretant TSH Ann Endocrinol (Paris) 33:390

Medeiros-Neto,G.A. 1977 T_3 thyrotoxicosis after iodinated contrast media Rev Paul Med 90:109

Nikolai,T.F.I. 1979:Lymphocytic thyroiditis with spontaneously resolving hyperthyroidism(silent thyroiditis)Thyroid Today 2(5):1-5

Steighiel,N.H.,Oppenheim,J.J.,Fisham,L.M.,Carbone,P.P. 1964 Metastatic embryonal carcinoma of the tests associated with elevated plasma TSH-like activity and hyperthyroidism New Engl j Med 271:345

Sung,L.C.,Cavalieri,R.R. T_3 Thyrotoxicosis due to metastatic thyroid carcinoma J Clin Endocrinol Metab 36:215

New Concepts in Thyroid Disease, pages 169–187

UNUSUAL MANIFESTATIONS IN PRIMARY HYPOTHYROIDISM

Kunihiro Yamamoto, Koshi Saito, Takaji Takai and Sho Yoshida
Department of Endocrinology and Metabolism,
Jichi Medical School,
Minamikawachi, Tochigi, Japan

The diagnosis of mild hypothyroidism has become easier with the recent development of radioimmunoassay. Thus, the clinical spectrum of hypothyroidism has broadened from subclinical hypothyroidism to full-blown myxedema. In more advanced hypothyroidism the chief complaints are esentially the same as in milder disease but more intense. By recent advancement in diagnosis tools, large amounts of information about the modifications that primary hypothyroidism develop in the physiology of main organs, has become available. We have focussed this study on the unusual manifestations of primary hypothyroidism; myocardial disfunction, respiratory disturbances, peripheral neuropathy and visual failure due to pituitary enlargement.

The aim of this study is to elucidate the prevalence of those manifestations in primary hypothyroidism which appear to be rather unusual (Watanakunakorn, C., 1965)

Materials and Methods

Nineteen patients with overt hypothyroidism (3 males and 16 females) with undetectable serum T_4 levels and high serum TSH levels were examined in this study. The mean duration of hypothyroidism was 8 years. Two patients became hypothyroid after subtotal thyroidectomy and one after radiation therapy for Graves' disease. Sixteen suffered idiopathic primary hypothyroidism presumably due to Hashimoto's thyroiditis. Antithyroid antibody tests (Fuzizoki, Japan) were positive in all patients.

1. Cardiovascular system. The cardiothoracic ratio was determined in a standard posteroanterior chest X-ray film. Myocardial function was evaluated by determination of systolic time intervals (Crowley, W. 1977). Total electromechanical systole ($Q-A_2$) and left ventricular ejection time (LVET) were measured directly, and the pre-ejection period (PEP) was calculated by subtraction ($PEP = Q-A_2 - LEVT$). PEP/LVET ratio was used as an index of myocardial contractility. The presence of pericardial effusion was examined using echocardiography. Subjects were scanned from apex to base. Pericardial effusion was diagnosed when the parietal and visceral layers of pericardium were clearly separated throughout both systole and diastole.

2. Respiratory system. Blood gas analyses at rest were performed in 13 patients with hypothyroidism. Arterial blood gases and pH were measured with a pH blood gas analyzer, and they were followed serially during thyroid hormone replacement therapy in 8 patients who had low arterial oxygen tension before therapy.

Ventilatory control was examined in 6 patients. Hypercapnic ventilatory drive was measured with the rebreathing technique. The subject rebreathed hyperoxic gas, and the linear relation between ventilation and alveolar carbon dioxide tension was evaluated as the slope of the response. In 2 patients with hypersomnolence and sleep apnea syndrome, the respiratory pattern was followed by spirogram recording during sleep. At the same time, arterial blood was drawn serially through a catheter which was indwelled into the radial artery.

3. Nervous system. Motor nerve conduction velocities were obtained in the ulnar, the median, the common peroneal and in the posterior tibial nerves by stimulating the nerves in appropriate places percutaneously and by obtaining compound muscle action potentials by surface electrodes. Sensory nerve conduction velocities were obtained in the ulnar, the median and in the sural nerves by anti-dromic stimulation. In the ulnar nerve 2 recording ring-shaped electrodes were placed on the fifth finger and in the median nerve on the index finger and stimulations were given percutaneously over the respective nerves at appropriate places in the elbow and the wrist. Thus, sensory nerve conduction velocities in the proximal segments (from the elbow to the wrist) and the distal segments (from the wrist to the fingers) were

calculated. In the sural nerve, stimulating electrodes were placed on the skin behind the external malleolus and the recording surface electrodes on the dorsum of the foot.

4. Visual function. The volume of the sella turcica was measured roentgenologically according to the method of Di Chiro and Nelson (1962). The 3 linear dimensions of the sella were obtained from routine lateral and posteroanterior roentgenograms of the skull. The visual field was determined by Goldmann's isopter perimetry. All patients with primary hypothyroidism were tested with the Goldmann's visual fields technique before and during thyroid hormone replacement therapy. Patients received TRH injection (500 ug intravenously) for the determination of peak TSH level. Total pituitary reserve of TSH was calculated by determining the total area under the curve for 120 min of this test.

Results

1. Cardiovascular system. The cardiothoracic ratio was determined in 19 patients with primary hypothyroidism. It was increased in 16 patients with ranges from 52 % to 72 %. Eighteen patients were examined for the presence of pericardial effusion using echocardiography. In 9 patients (50%), pericardial effusion was observed. A large effusion was observed in 2 patients who had high cardiothoracic ratios (72 % and 66 %). The cardiothoracic ratio, serum TSH level, age and the duration of hypothyroidism were compared between the 2 groups with and without pericardial effusion. The cardiothoracic ratio was significantly greater in the effusion positive group (effusion positive: 61.6 $\pm$ 5.1 %, effusion negative: 54.8 $\pm$ 5.8 %, $p<0.05$). But when patients who had excessive effusion were omitted, there was no significant difference between the two groups (effusion positive, 59.2 $\pm$ 3.2 %; effusion negative: 54.8 $\pm$ 5.8 %; N.S.). Cardiomegaly occurred in 7 of 9 patients in whom no pericardial effusion was demonstrable. The mean basal TSH level in effusion negative group was rather greater than that in positive group, but there was no difference between the two groups (effusion positive: 143.5 $\pm$ 71.8 uU/ml, effusion negative: 203.9 $\pm$ 99.4 uU/ml, N.S.). Neither the age of the patients nor the duration of the disease differed between the two groups.

Myocardial function was evaluated by determination of systolic time intervals using PEP/LVET ratio as an index of myocardial contractility. The mean value of PEP / LVET ratio in hypothyroidism was significantly greater than that in the control subjects (hypothyroidism: 0.55 $\pm$ 0.13, control: 0.32 $\pm$ 0.01, $p<0.001$). Grades of severity were classified as follows: mild change, 0.44 - 0.52; moderate, 0.53 - 0.60; marked, >0.60. Nine patients out of 12 (75 %) had increased PEP / LVET ratio (values over 0.44). Patients were divided into 2 groups according to the grade of severity in myocardial disfunction, PEP / LVET ratio over 0.53 and under 0.52. Patients with decreased myocardial contractility had significantly higher level of serum TSH (PEP / LVET >0.53 (n = 6 : 1683 $\pm$ 32.4 uU/ml, PEP / LVET <0.52 (n = 6): 104.6 $\pm$ 382 uU/ml, $p<0.01$). There was no significant correlation between the PEP / LVET ratio and grade of pericardial effusion. None of the parameters: cardiothoracic ratio, age and duration of primary hypothyroidism, correlated with PEP / LVET ratio. Patients were reassessed when they became euthyroid by thyroid hormone replacement therapy. All patients were improved by the therapy: the cardiac silhouette normalized, the pericardial effusion disappeared and the PEP / LVET ratio decreased to less than 0.44.

2. Respiratory system. Blood gas analyses were performed in 13 patients with hypothyroidism. Mean arterial oxygen saturation at rest was 92.8 %, mean P_aO_2 68.8 mmHg, mean P_aCO_2 412 mmHg and mean hematocrit 31.8 %. Nine patients had decreased arterial oxygen tension of under 70 mmHg. The incidence of hypoxia was 69 %. Two patients had increased arterial carbon dioxide tension of over 45 mmHg. There was no significant correlation between serum level of TSH and arterial oxygen tension or arterial carbon dioxide tension. Arterial blood studies were followed serially during thyroid hormone replacement therapy in 8 patients with decreased oxygen tension. Arterial oxygen tension increased and carbon dioxide tension decreased when the patients became euthyroid (P_aO_2; before: 61.6 $\pm$ 6.0, after: 78.9 $\pm$ 11.2 mmHg, $p< 0.005$, P_aCO_2; before: 42.0 $\pm$ 6.1, after: 35.6 $\pm$ 4.6 mmHg, $p <0.001$). Among 19 patients, 3 had hypersomnolence. Two of them also had sleep apnea syndrome. A nasal spirogram was recorded during sleep (Fig. 1). Observation of the patient during sleep revealed loud snoring. The end of the apneic periods was ushered by loud stridulous gasps. Cheyne-Stokes type respiration was observed when the patient seemed to be sleeping. The effective respirations were more regular than Cheyne-Stokes respiration. The periodic apnea was noted in spite of movement of the chest wall. The serial arterial gas

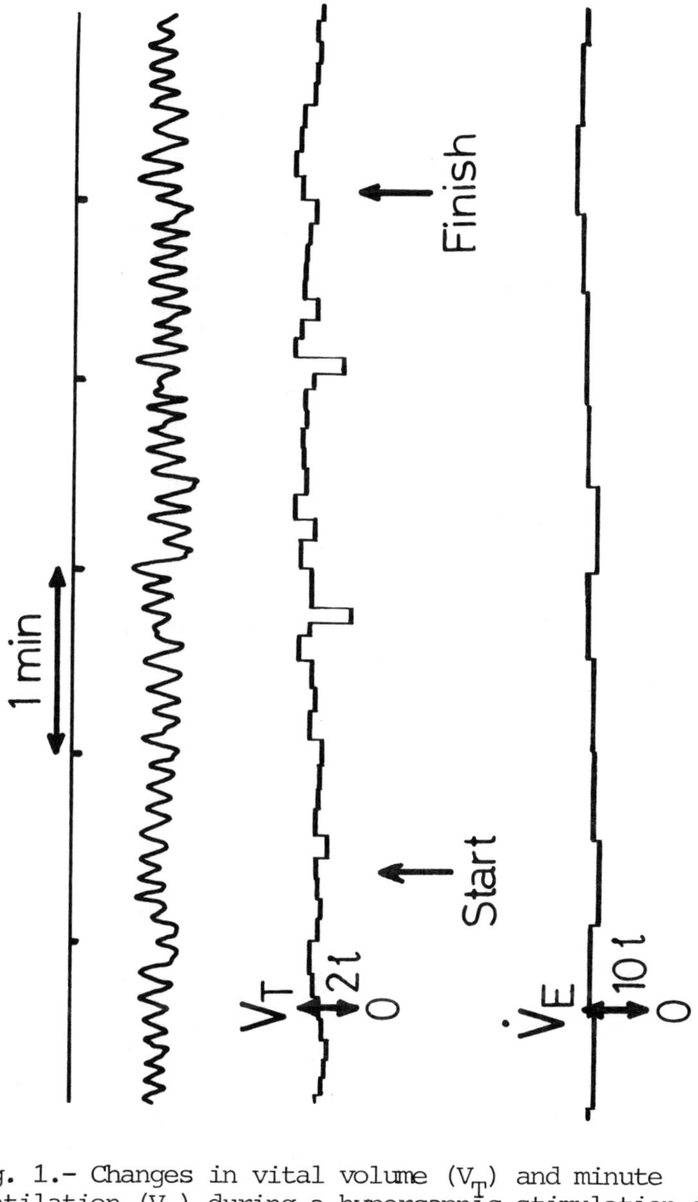

Fig. 1.- Changes in vital volume (V_T) and minute ventilation (V_E) during a hypercapnic stimulation in hypothyroidism. The respiratory pattern was followed by recording a nasal spirogram.

studies revealed decreased P_aO_2 and increased P_aCO_2 during sleep. In 6 patients examined with the ventilatory control, the index for hypercapnic ventilatory drive was lower than normal controls in all of them. After thyroid hormone replacement therapy, the index increased gradually but remained low (Fig. 2).

3. Nervous system. Fifteen patients were studied. Among them, only 2 had clinical manifestations of peripheral neuropathy. One patient had sensory symptoms alone and the other had both, motor and sensory symptoms. Mean conduction velocity in most of the motor nerves examined, showed a significant decrease in hypothyroidism compared to that in the control (Table 1). Distal latency showed significant prolongation in the median, the common peroneal and the posterior tibial nerves on both sides. The sensory nerves in the patients' distal segments (wrist to finger) of both ulnar and median nerves, showed significant decrease in conduction velocities compared to the control. However, the conduction velocity in the proximal segments (elbow to wrist) did not differ significantly from the controls.

Among the 11 patients in whom sensory nerve conduction studies were completed, 6 had values under the lower limits of our normal ranges in, at least, one of the sensory nerves examined. In the upper extremities these abnormalities were confined in the distal segments. Among the 15 patients who underwent motor nerve conduction studies, 6 had diminished values. However, in 2 of them, the decrease was only slight and was within normal limits when the age of the patients was considered. In 5 of these six, sensory nerves also showed diminished conductions. No motor weakness was noted in them. In one remaining patient unfortunately, studies on sensory nerves were not performed, although the patient had clinical manifestations of sensory-motor polyneuropathy.

4. Visual function. The roentgenographic measurements of the volume of the sella turcica were performed in 16 patients with primary hypothyroidism and 24 controls. The volume of the sella turcica was significantly enlarged in primary hypothyroidism when compared to that of controls (hypothyroid: 1173.1 ± 440.3 mm^3, control: 754.0 ± 145.9 mm^3, $p<0.01$). TSH level and total pituitary reserve of TSH correlated significantly with the volume of the sella turcica (Fig. 3 $r = 0.82$, $p < 0.001$).

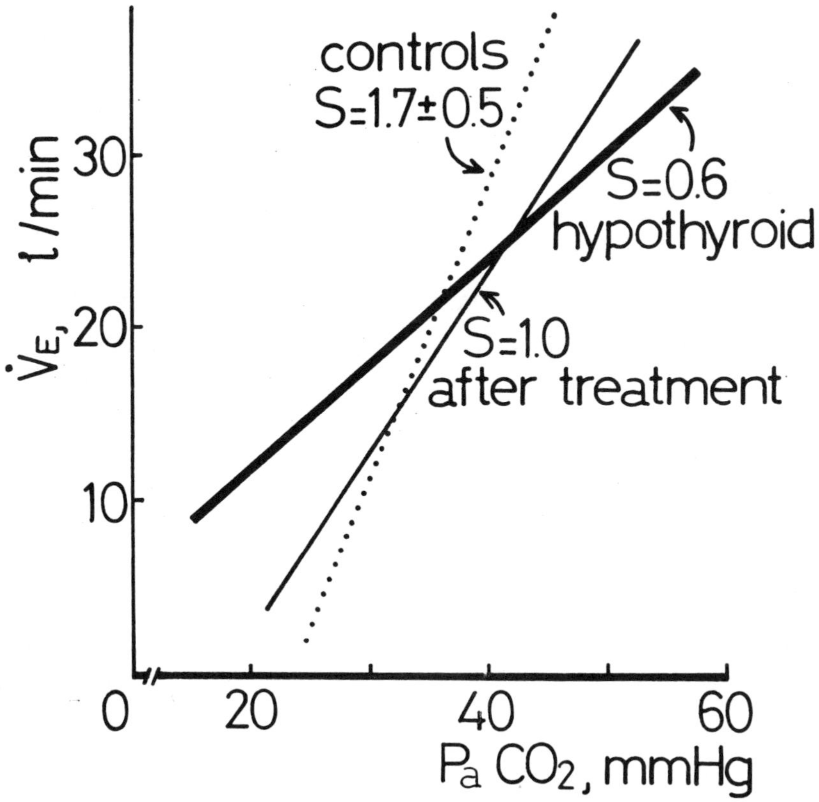

Fig. 2.- Ventilatory response in hypothyroidism. Hypercapnic ventilatory drive was studied as mentioned in Materials and Methods.

Fourteen patients with overt primary hypothyroidism were examined for the visual field by Goldmann's isopter perimetry. Visual fields in 10 patients were restricted. The prevalence was 71 % (Table 2). The grades of visual field defects distributed over a wide range, from an early sign of chiasmal compression to apparent bitemporal hemianopsia. Two patients complained of subjective visual failure, while 8 had no subjective symptoms. Figure 4 shows the mild changes of visual field defect in primary hypothyroidism. The abnormality in visual fields was characterized by the restriction in

TABLE 1
Motor and Sensory Nerve Conduction Velocities in Hypothyroidism

	Left	Right	Control (n=40)
Motor nerves (m/sec.)			
Ulnar	58.4 ± 4.2** (n=11)	62.0 ± 6.6 (n=10)	65.5 ± 4.9
Median	56.6 ± 5.9** (n=11)	55.0 ± 5.0** (n=10)	61.9 ± 4.9
Common peroneal	48.3 ± 4.3** (n= 9)	46.2 ± 3.8** (n=10)	54.3 ± 4.3
Posterior tibial	44.6 ± 3.6** (n=11)	44.6 ± 5.2* (n=10)	48.1 ± 3.3
Distal latencies (m/sec.)			
Ulnar	2.7 ± 0.6 (n=11)	2.7 ± 0.3 (n=10)	2.5 ± 0.4
Median	4.1 ± 1.0** (n=11)	4.1 ± 0.7** (n=10)	3.2 ± 0.7
Common peroneal	5.6 ± 1.0** (n= 9)	5.6 ± 1.2** (n=10)	4.6 ± 0.9
Posterior tibial	4.1 ± 1.0* (n=11)	4.0 ± 0.8* (n=10)	3.4 ± 0.7
Sensory nerves (m/sec.)			
Ulnar (wrist-finger)	47.6 ± 7.2** (n=10)	42.4 ± 4.7** (n= 6)	53.9 ± 5.6
Ulnar (elbow-wrist)	68.0 ± 4.4 (n=10)	64.8 ± 2.1 (n= 6)	67.5 ± 5.6
Median (wrist-finger)	48.3 ±11.0** (n=10)	44.9 ± 6.0** (n= 6)	56.3 ± 6.6
Median (elbow-wrist)	63.4 ± 5.3 (n=10)	61.9 ± 2.4 (n= 6)	63.8 ± 4.5
Sural	38.6 ± 6.8 (n= 7)	37.2 ± 5.2 (n= 5)	40.4 ± 4.4

mean ± standard deviation, **: $p < 0.01$, *: $p < 0.05$

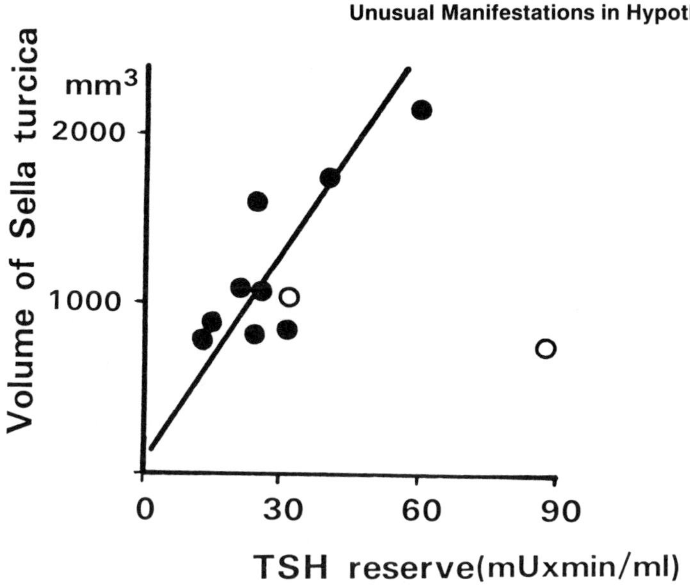

Fig. 3.- Correlation between the volume of the sella turcica and TSH reserve. The volume of the sella turcica and total pituitary TSH reserve were calculated as mentioned in Materials and Methods.

the central visual field while the peripheral visual field was less affected. In some cases, central scotoma was observed.

Ten patients with visual field defects were followed by serial examinations for Goldmann's visual field technique during thyroid hormone replacement therapy. Eight cases improved their restricted visual field after 1 - 4 months of therapy. In two cases, however, the visual field defect deteriorated during therapy. Figure 5 shows the time course of the change in visual field. Nasal lower quadrant anopsia in the right eye was observed before therapy. After 36 days of the replacement therapy, serum TSH level decreased to 60 uU/ml, but the patient complained that her visual failure took a bad turn. The Goldmann's visual field disturbance of this stage was aggravated to binasal lower quadrant anopsia. Thyroxine was increased to a dose of 200 ug/day. The visual

TABLE 2
Visual Field Defect in Primary Hypothyroidism

	Patients	Age	Sex	Duration	TSH (uU/ml)	Volume of Sella (mm^3)	Visual Field Defect	
1.	K.S.	39	F	13	336	760	(+)	(Subjective Sympt. (+) (Deterioration (+)
2.	K.Y.	62	M	10	86	891	(+)	Subjective Sympt. (+)
3.	N.O.	52	F	4	134	1064	(+)	Deterioration (+)
4.	C.A.	66	F	5	151	1755	(+)	
5.	T.W.	66	F	10	87	792	(+)	
6.	K.O.	42	F	4,5	148	1620	(±)	
7.	T.Mo.	58	F	6	133	1078	(±)	
8.	Y.F.	47	F	4,5	217	2150	(±)	
9.	S.K.	48	F	30	94	837	(±)	
10.	F.T.	50	F	5	342	1120	(±)	
11.	T.Ma.	58	F	3	127	1092	(−)	
12.	K.T.	38	M	3	183	1140	(−)	
13.	H.S.	44	F	4	152	850	(−)	
14.	T.H.	33	F	10	217	1920	(−)	

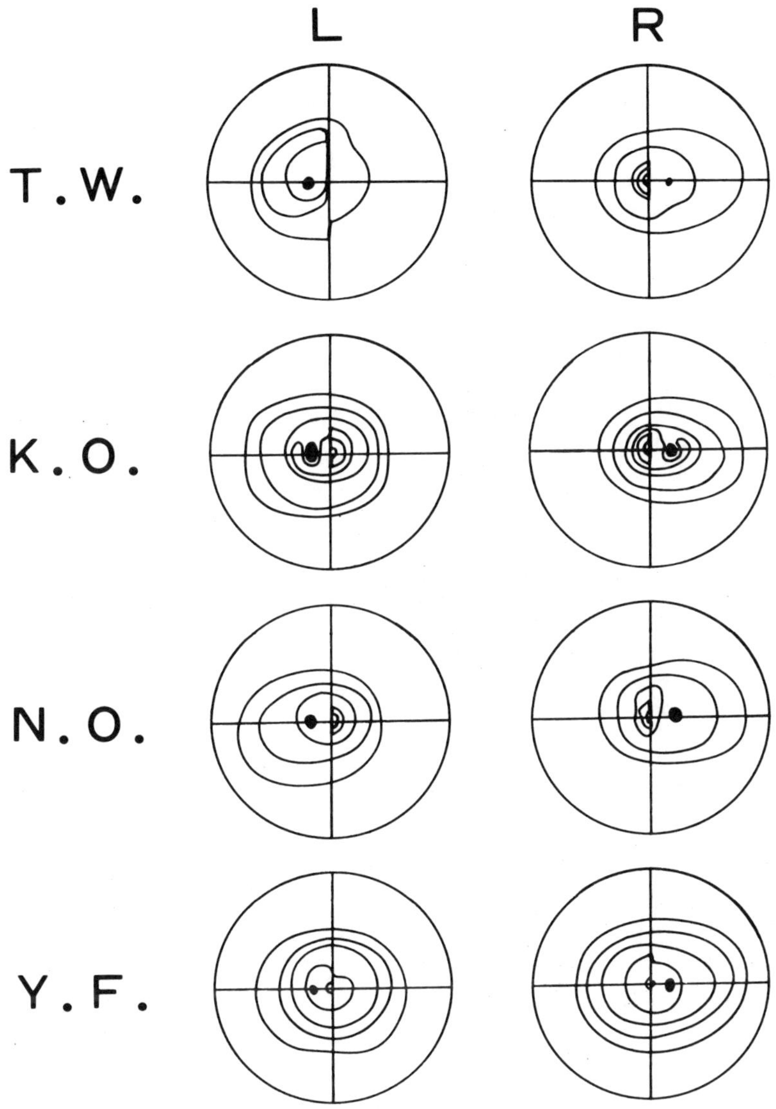

Fig. 4.- Minimal changes in visual failure in primary hypothyroidism. The visual field was examined with Goldmann's isopter perimetry.

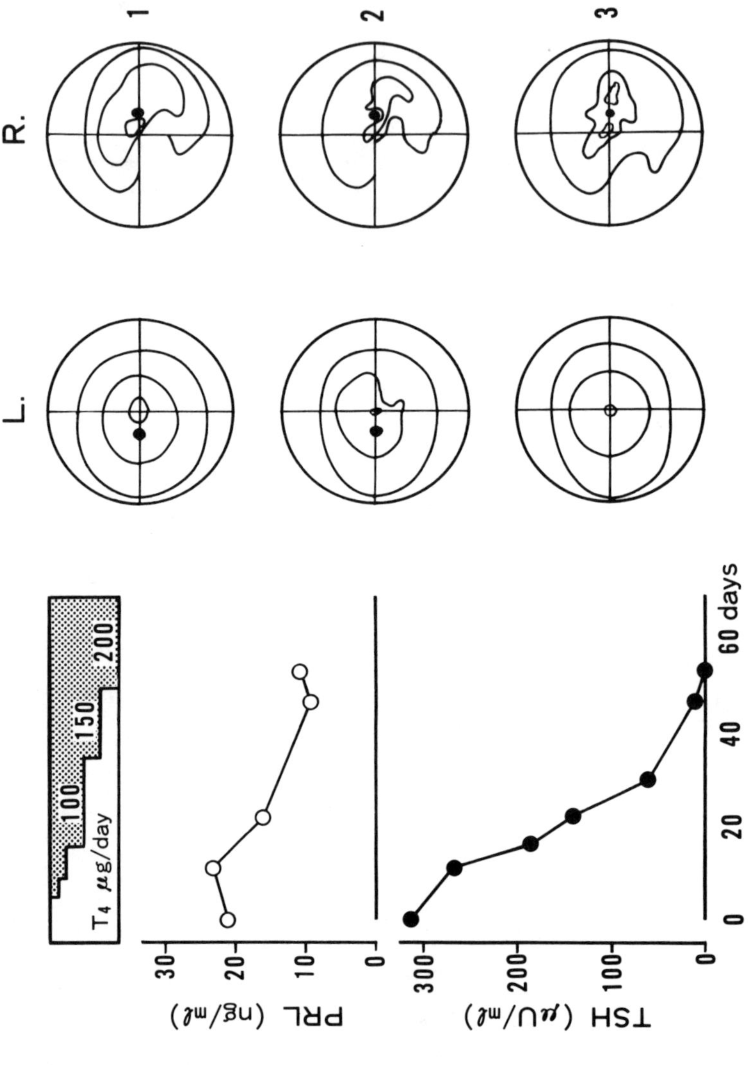

Fig. 5.- A deterioration of visual field defect during thyroid hormone replacement therapy. Visual fields: 1, before therapy; 2, on 36th day of therapy; 3, on 56th day of therapy.

field recovered when serum TSH was suppressed to undetectable levels. This patient also had galactorrhea. Her basal prolactin level was 22 ng/ml but increased to 310 ng/ml after TRH injection. Prolactin decreased during the replacement therapy and galactorrhea disappeared in spite of the fact that the patient complained of the deterioration in the visual failure. The time course of the deterioration in the visual failure in the other patient was followed. The visual field was restricted only in the central field before treatment. During the treatment with 100 ug thyroxine per day, the peripheral visual field restriction developed. The serum TSH level decreased from 134 uU/ml to 70 uU/ml. TRH stimulation test was performed before treatment and again at the time of the deterioration. The peak TSH level was higher after treatment than before treatment. The total pituitary TSH reserve did not decrease in spite of the thyroxine therapy (before: 30.3 mU·min/ml, after: 33.6 mU· min/ml). The visual field restriction improved when TSH level decreased to 2.6 uU/ml under prescription of thyroxine 150 ug/day.

Discussion

The aim of this study is to elucidate the prevalence of pericardial effusion, myocardial disfunction, respiratory disturbance, peripheral neuropathy and the visual failure in primary hypothyroidism. Among overt primary hypothyroidism 84 % of the patients had enlarged cardiac silhouette in the chest X-ray films. Under the examination by ultrasonography, 50 % of the patients had pericardial effusion. The patients with increased cardiothoracic ratio not necessarily had pericardial effusion.

Myocardial function was evaluated by determination of systolic time intervals. The PEP/LVET ratio has been demonstrated to correlate well with the cardiac output and stroke volume, and is usually used as an index of myocardial contractility.In 75 % of the patients, decreased myocardial function or moderate grade were observed. The grade of decreased myocardial function did not parallel with the grade of pericardial effusion. We confirmed the data of Crowley et al. that the PEP/LVET ratio closely parallels with the serum TSH level (Crowley, W., 1977). Severe myocardial disfunction may be present in overt hypothyroidism. In the cardiovascular manifestations of hypothyroidism, frequent incidence of low voltage complexes on the electrocardiogram had long before been recognized. The decreased myocardial contractility and the decline in the voltage on the electrocardiogram coincided well during the time course of the replacement therapy. Apparent increase in cardiac size in hypothyroidism may be due to pericardial effusion, myocardial disfunction or combination of both. This study indicates that roentgenographic cardiomegaly in hypothyroidism is rather rarely due to large pericardial effusion.

Alveolar hypoventilation may occur in hypothyroid patients who have no lung disease. Myxedema coma, a potentially lethal complication of hypothyroidism, is frequently associated with abnormalities of respiratory control. A high incidence of hypoxia was observed in this study which was not coincident with the data of Wilson and Bedell (1960). Hypoxia was improved by thyroxine replacement therapy along with the improvement of anemia. Existence of a depression of the respiratory center in the brain was suggested by the examination of ventilatory drive. The index of hypercapnic ventilatory drive was depressed in hypothyroidism.

Hypersomnolence was observed in 3 of 13 patients. Drowsiness during the day time was thought to be caused by by sleep disturbances. The sleep disturbance is known to be induced by the cyclic apnea. Further precise respiratory function test is needed to elucidate the mechanisms of hypoxia and the depression of the respiratory center in hypothyroidism.

Occurrence of peripheral neuropathy in hypothyroidism is well known (Meier, C., 1977). Carpal tunnel syndrome was also reported in hypothyroidism (Purnell, D., 1961). Presence of symmetric polyneuropathy was clearly demonstrated in this study. Although both motor and sensory nerves showed abnormal conduction in our study, most distinct involvement was seen in the distal segments of the sensory nerves. Unequivocal decrease of motor conduction was observed in only 4 of 15 patients. Prolongation of distal latency of motor nerves was seen in 8 of 15. The latter finding may be an early manifestation of motor nerve involvement; however, it can be taken as an unequivocal evidence of motor nerve lesion.

Abnormal nerve conduction velocities appear before clinical symptoms become manifest. In our series, only 2 patients had clinical symptoms in spite of the fact that 7 of 15 had a decrease in nerve conduction. Therefore, studies of nerve conduction velocities, particularly of the distal segments of the sensory nerves, seem to be a good screening test to rule out peripheral nerve involvement in hypothyroidism.

Pituitary enlargement owing to end-organ failure is not uncommon. Several reports have suggested that in some individuals, pituitary enlargement may be a secondary phenomenon, representing hyperplasia or adenomatous transformation of pituitary thyrotroph cells in response to primary hypothyroidism. Roentogenologic measurements of the volume of the sella turcica indicated an increase in primary hypothyroidism. The volume of the sella turcica closely related with the total pituitary TSH reserve. The data suggest that the increase in pituitary content of TSH may cause the pituitary enlargement in primary hypothyroidism. Since pituitary enlargement is not uncommon in primary hypothyroidism, a visual field defect as a sign of compression of the optic chiasm may appear repeatedly. Only 9 primary hypothyroid patients with visual failure have been reported in the literature (Skanse, B., 1956 - Saaman, N., 1977). Many cases reported showed a long lasting hypothyroidism before visual failure was noticed. Enlargement of the sella turcica was observed in all cases. Six cases had bilateral hemianopsia. For the treatment of the visual failure, 6 cases received thyroid hormone replacement therapy, 2 cases surgery and one case irradiation on the pituitary gland. Among 6 cases of thyroid hormone replacement therapy, 4 of them improved but 2 cases deteriorated their visual failure during the replacement therapy. The 2 patients with irreversible deterioration of visual failure suffered surgery for a pituitary tumor (Melnyk, C., 1965 - Stockigt, J., 1976). An unexpected high incidence of visual field defects was observed in our group. However, the abnormality of the visual field was rather mild. Only two patients complained of subjective visual failure. The visual field defects were characterized by a preferential lession in the central visual field as an early sign of chiasmal compression (Figure 3). It should be considered that over 90 % of the optic nerve really represents macular function (Kirkham, T., 1979). Thus, a compressive lesio of one optic nerve will always produce a central field defect. It is possible that the early signs of chiasmal compression may appear in the absence of the direct compression of optic chiasm. Bergland and Ray extensively studied on the blood supply of the optic chiasm (Bergland, R., 1969). The major supply to the central part of the chiasm that contains the crossing nasal fibers is from an inferior group of vessels of the vascular circle of Willis. The lateral part of the chiasm that contains the temporal, uncrossed visual fibers, is supplied by a superior and lateral group of vessels. Possibly, an expanding pituitary tumor first compresses the blood supply to the chiasm below thus causing visual field defect by creating a relative ischemia of the chiasm. Both ischemia and chiasmal direct compression are involved when the pituitary tumor enlarges enough. Ten patients with visual field defect were treated with thyroid hormone replacement therapy. In 2 patients, the visual field defect deteriorated during the replacement. The deterioration appeared when the serum TSH level decreased by 50% (Figure 5). When TSH stimulation test was performed, the peak TSH level was higher at the time of the deterioration than before treatment. The total pituitary TSH reserve did not differ in the two examinations. In an animal experiment, it is reported that the administration of a small dose of thyroxine to hypothyroid rat induced an enlargement of pituitary gland along with an increase in pituitary TSH content (D'Angelo, S., 1969). The possible mechanism of the paradoxical pituitary enlargement may be as follows: In primary hypothyroidism, synthesis and release of TSH by the anterior pituitary gland are accerated under the stimulation of TRH. Thyroid hormone may have separate effects on the synthesis and release of TSH. Both mechanisms may be inhibited by thyroid hormone but the thresholds may differ. Low dosage of thyroid hormone may suppress the release of TSH but not the synthesis. Thus, pituitary TSH content may increase. Sufficient dosage of thyroid hormone may suppress both release and synthesis of TSH, and the pituitary TSH content decrease. The size of the pituitary gland is supposed to be parallel with the TSH content. Two cases with deteriorated visual failure in the previous literature were treated by surgery. In our experiences, it is feasible to treat such patients with deteriorated visual failure with thyroid hormone replacement therapy, under a careful follow up study for the visual field. The improvement in the deteriorated visual field defect with hyperreplacement dosage of thyroid hormone, suggests that the visual failure is caused by the pituitary hypertrophy rather than the pituitary tumor.

In brief; Unexpected high incidence of the unusual manifestations was observed. Since we used sensitive tools for detection, subclinical signs were found in this study.

It is suggested that the manifestations which are thought to be rare may appear when the patient has already fallen down to hypothyroidism although its grade is less intense.

Abstract

Nineteen patients with overt hypothyroidism were examined for the prevalence of myocardial disfunction, respiratory disturbances, peripheral neuropathy, and visual failure due to pituitary enlargement. Prevalences of pericardial effusion and myocardial disfunction (decrease PEP/LVET) were 50% and 75%, respectively. The degree of decreased myocardial function did not parallel with the grade of pericardial effusion.

Arterial blood analysis indicated a frequent incidence of hypoxia in hypothyroidism. The incidence of hypoxia was 69%. The hypoxia was improved by thyroxine replacement therapy. In 6 patients examined for the ventilatory control, all had the index for hypercapnic ventilatory drive lower than normal control. It was suggested that the hypoxia in hypothyroidism was caused by a depression of the respiratory center in the brain and by anemia.

Sensory nerve conduction was diminished in 6 of 11 hypothyroid patients and motor conduction in 6 of 15 was studied. In distal segments of sensory nerves, the abnormality frequently appeared before clinical symptoms of polyneuropathy.

Visual field defect was detected in 71% of patients suffering of primary hypothyroidism. The most common characteristic change was the defect in the central visual field. All cases of visual field defect were cured by thyroid hormone replacement therapy. Two cases with deteriorated visual failure who did not improve during physiological replacement, were successively treated with over dosage of thyroid hormone.

ACKNOWLEDGEMENTS

Supported in part by a research grant for "Special Diseases" of the Japanese Ministry of Health and Welfare

REFERENCES

Balsam, A., Oppenheimer, J.H., 1975 Pituitary tumor with primary hypothyroidism N Y St J Med 75:1737
Bergland, R., Ray, B.S., 1969 The arterial supply of the human optic chiasm. J Neurosurg 31:327
Caughey, J.E., Lester, M.J., Hypothyroidism and pituitary tumours. NZ Med J 60:486
Crowley, W.F., Ridgway, E.C., Bough, E.W., Francis, G.S., Daniels, G.H., Kourides, I.A., Myers, G.S., Maloof, F., 1977 Noninvasive evaluation of cardiac function in hypothyroidism. N Engl J Med 296:1
D'Angelo, S.A., 1969 Action of target gland hormones on pituitary TSH rebound: Variation of the threshold hypothesis of TSH secretion.
Di Chiro, G., Nelson, K.B., 1962 The volume of the sella turcica Am J Roentgenol Radium Ther Nucl Med 87:989
Kirkham, T.H., 1979 Neuroophthalmology: Clinical assessment of visual function. Signs and symptoms of pituitary tumours. Clinical Neuroendocrinology: A Pathophysiological Approach, (edited by G. Tolis, et al.). Raven Press, New York p 385
Leiba, S., Landau, B., Ber, A., 1960 Target gland insufficiency and pituitary tumours Acta Endocrinol 60:112
Meier, C., Bischoff, A., 1977 Polyneuropathy in Hypothyroidism J Neurol 215:103
Melnyk, C.S., Greer, M.A., 1965 Functional pituitary tumor in an adult possibly secondary to long-standing myxedema. J Clin Endocrinol 25:761
Nagai, K., Nagata, K., 1976 A case of chronic thyroiditis with enlargement of sella turcica and a chiasmal syndrome Kansai denryoku byoin igakuzashi 8:123 (in japanese)
Purnell, D.C., Daly, D.D., Lipscomb, P.R., 1961 Carpal-tunnel syndrome associated with myxedema. Arch Intren Med 108:751
Stockigt, J.R., Essex, W.B., West, R.H., Murray, R.M.L., Breidahl, H.D.,1976 Visual failure during replacement therapy in primary hypothyroidism with pituitary enlargement. J Clin Endocrinol Metab 43:1094
Skanse, B., Aren, A., 1956 Disappearance of bi-temporal hemianopsla following correction of myxedema in a case of chromophobe pituitary tumour. Acta Endocrinol 23:289
Saaman, N.A., Osborne, B.M., Mackay, B., Leavans, M.E., Duello, T.M., Halmi, N.S., 1977 Endocrine and morphologic studies of pituitary adenomas secondary to primary hypothyroidism. J Clin Endocrinol Metab 45:903
Vagenakis, A.G., Dole, K., Braverman, L.E., 1976 Pituitary

enlargement, pituitary failure, and primary hypothyroidism Ann Intern Med 85:195
Watanakunakorn, C., Hodges, R.E., Evans, T.C., 1965 Myxedema A study of 400 cases. Arch Intern Med 116:183
Wilson, W.R., Bedell, G.N., 1960 The pulmonary abnormalities in myxedema. J. Clin Invest 39:42

New Concepts in Thyroid Disease, pages 189–205

DIAGNOSIS OF EXOPHTHALMOS USING ORBITAL ULTRASONOGRAPHY AND TREATMENT OF MALIGNANT EXOPHTHALMOS WITH STEROID THERAPY, ORBITAL RADIATION THERAPY, AND PLASMAPHERESIS

Kunihiro Yamamoto, Koshi Saito, Takaji Takai and Sho Yoshida
Department of Endocrinology and Metabolism, Jichi Medical School, Minamikawachi, Tochigi, Japan

The existence of a unique type of ophthalmopathy in hyperthyroidism was described about 200 years ago. The association of thyroid disfunction with appearance of eye symptoms was first described by Parry in 1786. In spite of a vast amount of investigation about eye changes in Graves' disease, the pathogenesis of this disorder remains obscure. The diagnosis of Graves' ophthalmopathy is usually not a clinical problem, but evaluation of the precise location and extent of intraorbital changes leaves much to be elucidated. The most severe manifestation, malignant exophthalmos, is often encountered in patients who become euthyroid or hypothyroid during therapy for hypothyroidism, but there is no satisfactory method to predict the outcome or severity of the exophthalmos in these individuals

To verify the intraorbital changes in Graves' disease and to establish a quantitative analysis of the extraocular muscle changes, we used B-mode ultrasonography as a non-invasive procedure.

Many therapeutic approaches to malignant exophthalmos have been proposed, but although each therapy has been reported to offer effective results, none of them gained a wide acceptance so as to be regardedas a standard method of therapy. We have treated 7 patients with moderately severe ophthalmology due to Graves' disease with corticosteroid therapy, supervoltage orbital radiotherapy and plasmapheresis. The results of each therapy were compared.

MATERIALS AND METHODS

I. Diagnosis of Exophthalmos

1.Eye protrusion in patients with Graves' disease. Proptosis was examined in 113 patients with Graves' disease and in 140 patients with euthyroid diabetes mellitus as controls.The proptosis was measured with a Hertel type exophthalmometer.The measurements were carried out by one observer using one Hertel' sexophthalmometer to minimize the erros in measurements.

2.Ultrasonography of the orbital soft tissue.Both orbits of thirty one patients with Graves' disease were studied. Seventeen were untreated and fourteen were on treatment with antithyroid drugs,but not in remission.Six euthyroid diabetic patients with negative thyroid autoantibody tests were assessed as controls.All patients investigated in this study had no signs or symyoms of ophthalmopathy except proptosis.Proptosis in the group was distributed over a range between 13mm and 23mm.Equipments for ultrasonographic diagnostic set were Aloka-SSD-60B and an opthalmoscanner, MSU-12B.A 5 MHZ transducer,13mm in diameter,with a 5.5mm focal pint was used.Horizontal scanning was accomplished in a position permiting the apraisal of the maximal diameter in both eyes.

3.Quantitative evaluation of the extraocular muscles. A map of the image was depicted on paper.The distance between the lateral orbital wall and the intraorbital fat was measured in mm and the value represented the "muscle index".The details of the measurements are indicated elsewhere (Yamamoto,K. 1979).The muscle index is supposed to indicate the diameter of the lateral rectus muscle.

4.Assay of TSI,thyroglobulin and acid mucopolysaccharide. Thyroid stimulating immunoglobulins (TSI) activities were assayed in 30 patients with Graves' disease including 6 patients with malignanr exophthalmos.The assay method was essentially the same as described by Smith and Hall(1974). A crude fraction of human thyroid membrane was collected from thyroid tissue of Graves' disease according to the method of Manley et al(1974).Rat TSH,obtained from Dr.Palow, NIH,was radioiodinated by chloramine T method and used as the tracer.Immunoglobulin was fractionated by ammonium sulfate and the amount of 2mg/tube was used.B/F separation was performed using polyethylene glycol.

Serum thyroglobulin concentrations were measured by the method of Van Herle (1973).Twenty-two patients with untreated Graves' disease with negative anti-thyroglobulin antibody test (Fuzi Zoki,Japan) were chosen for the measurement.Since serum thyroglobulin level in Graves' patients is known to decreas during antithyroid drug therapy (Uller,R.,1978) patients under this treatment were omitted.

Serum level of acid mucopolysaccharide was assayed by the method of Winand (1968).Acid mucopolysaccharide was extracted from 2ml serum samples and measured by spectrophotometry after cabazol reaction.Sera from 24 patients with Graves' disease and 5 control subjects were assayed.

II.Treatment of Malignant Exophthalmos

Several patients with malignant exophthalmos (4 males, 3 females) were treated with steroid therapy,supervoltage orbital radiotherapy or plasmapheresis.Six patients with moderately severe ophthalmopathy due to Graves' disease were treated with steroid therapy and supervoltage orbital radiotherapy succesively.One patient with corneal ulceration was treated with plasmapheresis.All patients complained of chemosis,ocular pain and diplopia.The mean value for proptosis in the patients was 21.5mm(ranging between 18and 23mm). The mean value for the muscle index was 8.1 which was more than twice that of controls.

1.<u>Steroid therapy</u>.a.Systemic glucocorticoid therapy-Prednisolone 100mg/day was prescribed in 3 patients for two weeks and the outcome of the therapy was followed for 4 weeks.

b.Retrobulbar injection of glucocorticoid-Other 3 patients were treated with retrobulbar injection of 20mg of methylprednisolone acetate(depot type) once a week for 4-5 weeks.The outcome of the therapy was followed for 4 weeks after the retrobulbar injection.

2.<u>Supervoltage orbital radiotherapy</u>.Radiotherapy was performed with the method described by Donaldson et al.(1973). A finely collimated beam delivered from supervoltage linear accelerator was used.A fractionated dose of 2,000 rads was delivered over 10 days,Monday through Friday in two consecutive weeks.The outcome of therapy was followed for at least 6 months.

3.<u>Plasmapheresis</u>.A patient with Graves' disease and malignant exophthalmos was treated with plasmapheresis.The patient had manifest exophthalmos (Hertel reading:right eye, 21mm;left eye,19mm),diplopia and ulceration of cornea.Four sessions of plasma exchange were performed using an Haemonetics cell separator.About 5 L of plasma were exchanged for the same volume of normal fresh-frozen plasma and saline Immunosuppression was also carried out with prednisolone(60 mg/day).The cell separator enabled us to draw blood,separate plasma fraction and return the cellular fraction of blood with normal fresh-frozen plasma,continuously.Blood was drawn at a rate of 30-40ml/min and 1 L of plasma was exchanged within 90 min.

4.Evaluation of the effect of the therapy.The effect of the therapy was judged by scoring the opthalmopathy index (Donaldson,S.S.,1973)due to the classification of the signs and symptoms of exophthalmos by Werner (1977).Scores for the proptosis were modified to fit the degrees of proptosis in Japanese(minimal (1):16-19mm,moderate(2):19-22mm,marked(3): >22mm)which is less than that in Caucasians

Results

Protrusion of the eyes in the patients with Graves' disease.The mean value of Hertel reading was 14.1mm in control subjects,while Graves' patients had larger mean value of 17.1mm.Proptosis in Graves' disease was significantly increased beyond normal by about 3mm (Table 1).

Table 1. Protrusion in Graves' disease and controls

		Hertel reading (mm)
Graves' disease	(113)	17.09± 2.79*
Controls	(140)	14.10± 2.64

*$p < 0.001$

Ultrasonography of the orbital soft tissue in Graves' disease.An image of the orbits in normal controls is shown in Figure 1.As illustrated bellow in the figure,medial and lateral orbital walls and intraorbital fat are defined. The space between the orbital walls and the intraorbital fat represents the medial and lateral rectus muscles.Orbital image in one Graves' patients showed swelling of the lateral and medial rectus muscles (Fig. 1).This is the minimal change of extraocular muscles in Graves' disease and this patient had no clinical signs or symtoms of exophthalmos.The muscle index,as a parameter of the diameter of lateral rectus muscle, was measured in the tracing map of the ultrasonographic image as reported before(Smith,B.,1974).The muscle index in

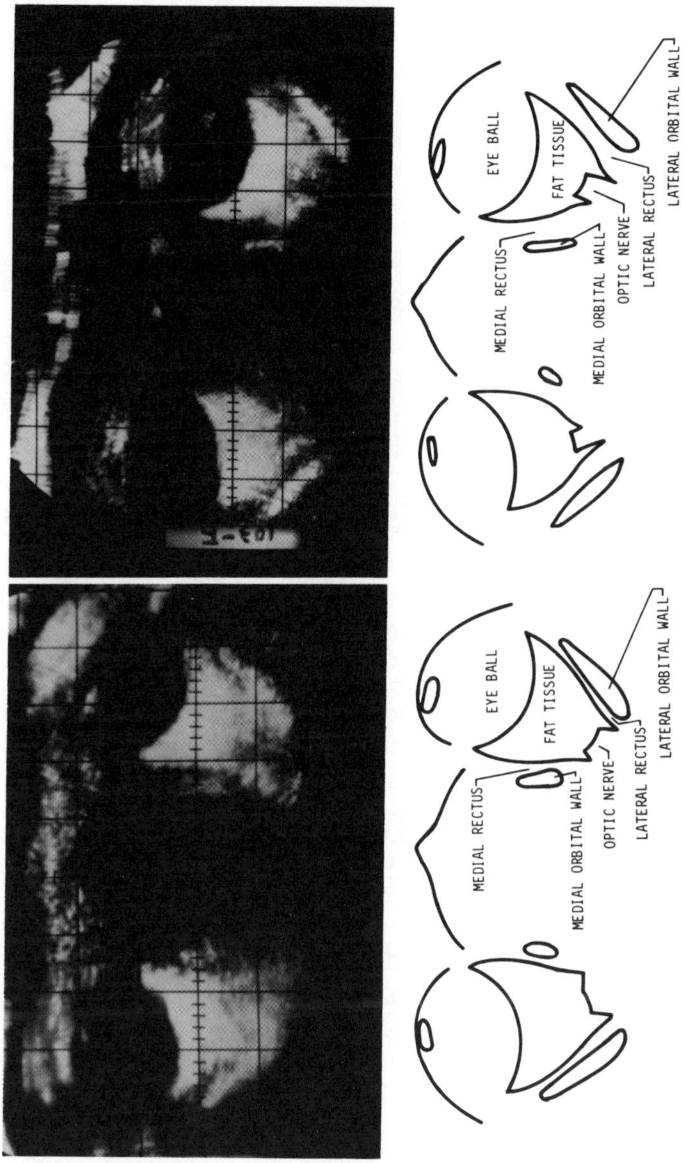

Fig.1-An ultrasonographic image of the orbits. (left)Normal orbits.(right)Orbits in Graves' patient showing the swelling of the lateral and medial rectus muscles.

Graves' disease was significantly larger than that of control subjects(Table 2).The subjects were divided into 4 groups based on the degree of the ocular protrusion (Group I, control subjects with Hertel reading 13-15mm;Group II Graves' patients with Hertel reading 13-15 mm;Group III Graves' patients with Hertel reading 16-18mm;Group IV Graves'patients with Hertel reading more than 18mm).The muscle index value in the 4 groups were compared (Fig 2).The control subjects had a mean value of 3.10.The Graves' patients with the same degree of proptosis (Group II) as the control subjects had the mean value of 4.62 which was significantly increased.The muscle index increased as the degree of proptosis increased in Graves' patients (Group I:3.10 ± 1.29,Group II:4.62 ± 2.29, Group III:6.34 ± 1.68,Group IV:7.72 ± 3.42).The muscle index correlated significantly with Hertel's reading (Fig.3).Some patients without proptosis had increased muscle index values of over 3.10.

Thyroid stimulating immunoglobulin(TSI),thyroglobulin and acid mucopolysaccharide in the serum in Graves' disease (Table II).Immunoglobulins from Graves' patients inhibited the binding of TSH to human thyroid membrane fraction. TSI activity was positive in 76.7% of Graves' patients. Patients with Graves' disease were divided into 3 groups according to the muscle index.There was no significant correlation between TSI index and the degree of extraocular muscle enlargement.

Serum thyroglobulin level increases in untreated Graves' patients compared with control subjects.There was no significant correlation between the serumlevel of thyroglobulin and the degree of extraocular muscle enlargement.

Contents of acidmucupolysaccharide in the sera from Graves' patients increased significantly compared with 5 control sera,but no correlation was observed between the acid mucupolysaccharide concentration and the degree of the extraocular muscle changes.

Treatment of malignant exophthalmos.Every patient who received steroid therapy showed some improvement in ocular pain,chemosis and diplopia.The ophthalmopathy index decreased significantly after therapy (Table 3).One patient who received systemic glucocorticoid therapy decreased his proptosis(from 18 to 15mm)along with a marked improvement in soft tissue involvement.His clinical remission continued for more than 3 years after the steroid therapy was finished.In other five patients who received steroid therapy,no improvement in proptosis or extraoculas muscle enlargement was observed by means of an ultrasonogram of the orbit.These patients

TABLE 2

Thyroid stimulating immunoglobulin(TSI),thyroglobulin(Tg) and acid mucopoly saccharide (AMPS) in the serum of Graves' disease.

	TSI index	Tg (mg/ml)	AMPS (mg/dl)
Control	101.8 ± 6.6 (6)	6.8 ± 2.3(8)	280 0 ± 40.8(5)
Graves' disease	71.8 ± 19.9 (30)**	189.4 ± 46.2(22)***	662.9 ± 304.2(24)*
Muscle index			
~5.0	68.5 ± 19.8 (9)	212.6 ± 123.9 (9)	642.0 ± 306.8 (5)
5.0~6.5	75.0 ± 20.0 (13)	240.8 ± 119.5 (10)	682.7 ± 360.8 (11)
6.5~	70.1 ± 21.7 (8)	139.3 (3)	648.8 ± 251.0 (8)

* $P < 0.01$, ** $P < 0.005$, *** $P < 0.001$

Assays of TSI index,serum thyroglobulin and serum acid mucupolysaccharide were performed as indicated in Materials and Methods.
Graves' patients were divided into 3 groups according to theis muscle index.

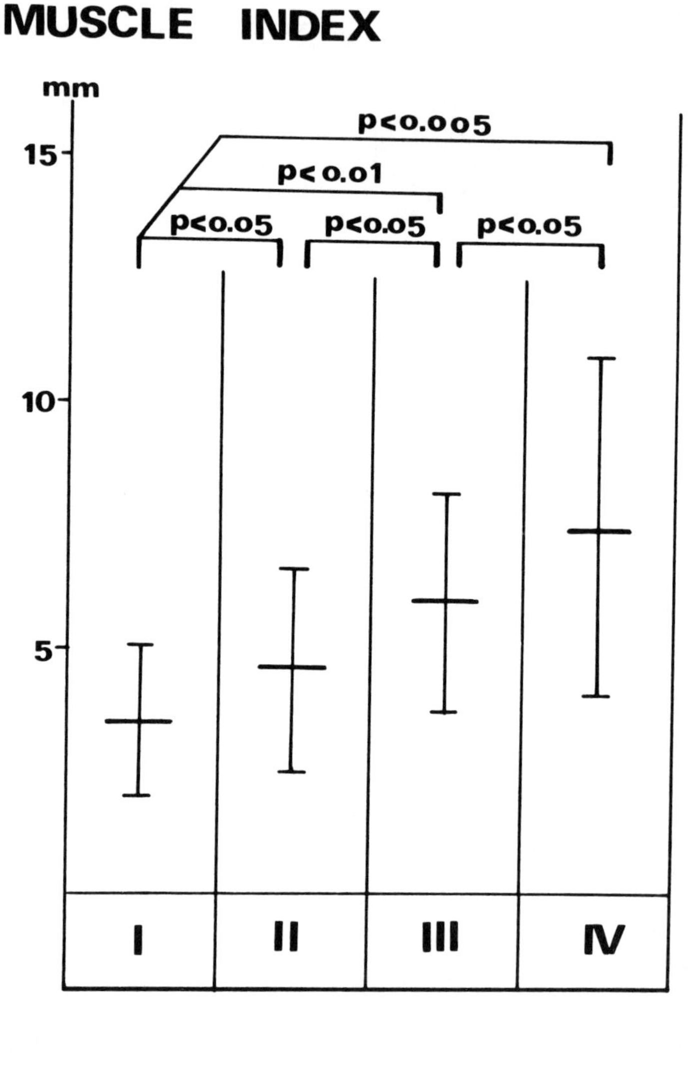

Fig.2 Changes in the muscle index in Graves' disease.The muscle index was calculated as mentioned in Materials and Methods.The groups I - IV were divided as indicated in the text.

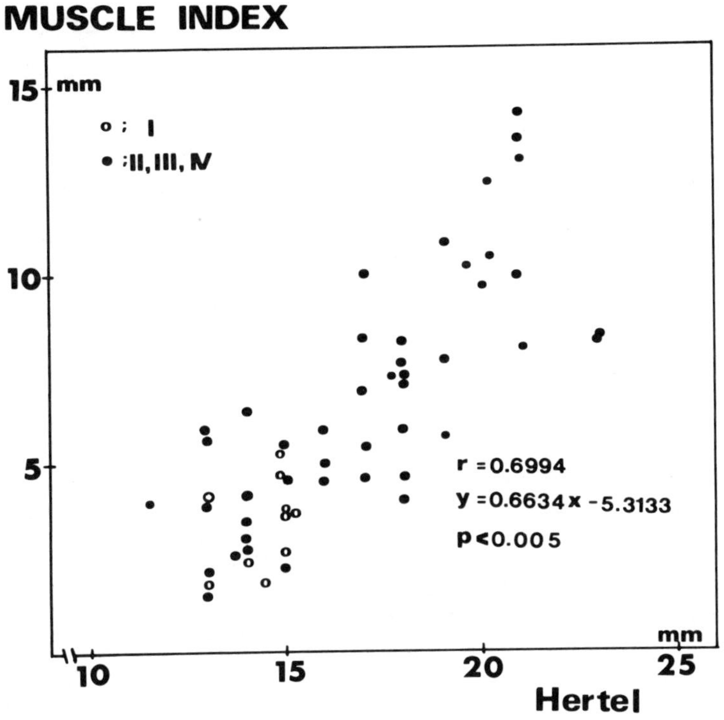

Fig.3 The correlation between proptosis and the muscle index.The muscle index was calculated as mentioned in Materials and Methods.

received succesive radiation therapy for treatment of proptosis.

TABLE 3 Changes in ophthalmopathy index by the steroid and orbital radiation therapy for malignant exophthalmos.

		Ophthalmopathy index	
Steriod therapy (6)	before	4.7 ± 1.5	$p < 0.005$
	after	2.5 ± 1.5	
Orbital radiation (5) therapy	before	2.8 ± 1.5	N.S.
	after	1.4 ± 0.6	

Ophthalmopathy index was calculated as mentioned in Materials and methods. Number of the patients is indicated in parenthesis.

Orbital radiation therapy significantly decreased proptosis in these patients when compared with the value before treatment. (Table 4). It should be noticed that the Hertel' s reading after radiation therapy was still greater than that in Graves' patients without infiltrative ophthalmopathy. The same results were obtained with the orbital radiation therapy when we examined the changes in the extraocular muscle enlargement. The müscle index decreased significantly with this therapy, but after radiation therapy it was still greater than that in Graves' disease without infiltrative ophthalmopathy (Table 5). The beneficial effect of steroid therapy on the symptoms of the orbital soft tissue involvement, (ocular pain, chemosis, epiphora, and diplopia) appeared only after 3 to 4 weeks of therapy. On the other hand the improvement in proptosis after the orbital radiation therapy appeared after 3-7 months of therapy.

Serum levels of acid mucopolysaccharide were measured in 3 patients with malignant exophthalmos, before and after steroid and orbital radiation therapy. Serum level decreased in 2 patients who decreased the muscle index by more than 2, but did not change in one patient who only had a minimal change in the muscle index.

TABLE 4. Changes in proptosis by the orbital radiation therapy

	Hertel reading (mm)	
before therapy (5)	21.5 ± 1.7	$p < 0.005$
after therapy (5)	19.2 ± 1.8	$p < 0.02$
Graves' patients without infiltrative ophthalmopathy (11)	16.7 ± 2.9	

The regimen of the orbital radiation therapy is indicated in Materials and Methods. Number of the patients is indicated in parenthesis.

TABLE 5. Changes in the muscle index by the steroid and orbital radiation therapy

	Muscle index	
before therapy (6)	8.1 ± 1.8	$p < 0.005$
after therapy (6)	6.9 ± 1.7	$p < 0.05$
Graves' patients without infiltrative ophthalmopathy (10)	5.2 ± 1.0	$p < 0.05$
Control (12)	3.4 ± 1.5	

The muscle index was calculated as mentioned in Materials and Methods. The therapy regimes are indicated in Materials and Methods. Number of the patients is indicated in parenthesis.

The effect of plasmapheresis was much more precocious when compared to the steroid therapy and supervoltage orbital radiotherapy. Changes in proptosis and ophthalmopathy index during and after plasmapheresis are shown in Figure 4. At the end of the fourth session of plasma exchange, proptosis decreased by 2mm and ulceration of the cornea recovered, double vision also improved subjectively and the ophthalmopathy index decreased from 7 to 2.During the tapering of prednisolone,double vision and chemosis were aggravated with a noticeable increase in exophthalmos.The patient was re-admitted and plasmapheresis restarted.By 3 sessions of plasmapheresis,chemosis disappeared,double vision and exophthalmos improved.There were no serious complications except hypotension which occurred at the first session of the first plasma exchange.Serum immune complex concentrations were measured by enzyme immunoassay using $C1_q$ as complement.Levels decreased in parallel with the improvement of symptoms although serum concentration was originally within normal range.(Table 6).

TABLE 6.Changes in immune complex level during plasmapheresis

	Immune complex (ug/ml)
1st plasmapheresis	
before	3.0
after	2.1
2nd plasmapheresis	
before	2.6
after	2.0

The regimen of plasmapheresis is indicated in Materials and Methods.

Discussion

In a large random sample of patients with Graves' disease,ocular protrusion was found to be increased beyond normal by about 3mm.These data suggest that almost all patients with Graves' disease have exophthalmos.It is impossible that ocular protrusion of about 3mm may be found in most patients in whom no exophthalmos is diagnosed clinically.The presence of uniform enlargement of the extraocular muscles in Graves' disease was also indicated by ultrasonographic studies of the orbital soft tissue.The muscle index in Graves' patients without clinical signs of exophthalmos (Hertel reading 13-15mm)increased significantly when compared with the control subjects,although both groups had the same degree of proptosis(Fig.2).When the muscle index and the Hertel reading were compared there was a significant positive correlation(Fig 3).The data indicate

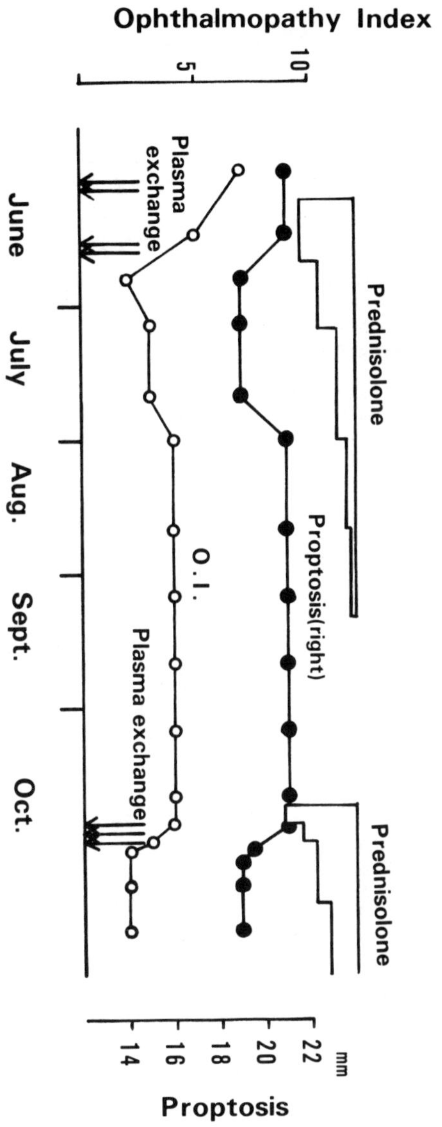

Fig.4-The changes in proptosis and ophthalmopathy index during plasmapheresis.The details of the patient profile and the method of the therapy are indicated in Materials and Methods.

that the muscle index is a reliable parameter of extraocular muscle change.Also,the data suggest that even the smallest increase in the bulk of the orbital tissue may cause some ocular protrusion.

Since almost all patients with Graves' disease might have extraocular muscle enlargement,it is suggested that the same pathogenetic factor may play a role in hyperthyroidism and exophthalmos in Graves' disease.We examined the serum levels of TSI,thyroglobulin and acid mucopolysaccharide in this group of Graves' patients.None of the factors correlated with the extraocular muscle changes which were assessed by ultrasonography.Acid mucupolysaccharide is reported to be related with the intraorbital changes in Graves' disease(Winand,R.I.,1968).The absence of correlation in our data may be due to the moderate changes of ophthalmopathy in the subjects studied.During the course of therapy for malignant exophthalmos,acid mucupolysaccharide content was decreased in 2 patients with some clinical improvement of exophthalmos.It is possible that the acid mucupolysaccharide content may parallel the degree of exophthalmic changes if exophthalmos in Japanese is as severe as in Caucasians.

Among the Graves' patients with exophthalmos,those with progressive symptoms beyond class 2 (Werner,S.C.,1977)may need treatment.Many therapeutic approaches to malignant exophthalmos have been reported,but ,up to now,none of them has gained wide acceptance so as to be regarded as a standard method for therapy.Reports of Donaldson et al.(1973)and Covington et al.(1977)suggested that the supervoltage orbital radiotherapy was a very effective and safe method. Nevertheless,very recently,Teng et al.(1980) reported that the supervoltage orbital radiotherapy is not so effective, at least in the patients with moderately severe ophthalmopathy.From the analysis of our results the supervoltage orbital radiotherapy is not sufficiently effective.The Hertel reading after the therapy was still greater than that in Graves' patients without infiltrative ophthalmopathy (Table 4),although the proptosis in the patients with infiltrative ophthalmopathy decreased significantly by the supervoltage orbital radiotherapy.None of the patients under the orbital radiotherapy returned their eye globes to normal position.The maximal improvement in proptosis appeared after 3-7 months.In previous reports the supervoltage orbital radiotherapy was characterized by their early effects which appeared within 3 months in the early stage of the therapy. In our experience,the improvements in the soft tissue involvement appeared after 3-4 weeks of the steroid or radiation thaerapy.But the effects in proptosis appeared gradually during 3-7 months after the radiation therapy.

The effects of the radiation therapy should be judged after 6 months of therapy.A rapid improvement in proptosis was observed during plasma exchange therapy,but the effect was transient and the symptoms of exophthalmos regained after a short period of remission.

The data of our series of therapy indicate the following lines:

1.Both steroid therapy and orbital radiation therapy are effective for the symptoms of orbital soft tissue involvement such as ocular pain,epiphora,chemosis and lid swelling and for diplopia.

2.All patients treated with supervoltage orbital radiation therapy diminish their exophthalmos and the improvement is maintained for over 18 months,but the improvement in proptosis appears only after 3-7 months after therapy

3.Plasmapheresis is an effective method of therapy for malignant exophthalmos especially in the acute phase of the disease.Compared with the effect of radiation therapy,the effect of plasmapheresis appears rapidly after therapy

4. To maintain the acute effect of plasmapheresis, combination of immunosuppression therapy such as steroid and /or orbital radiation therapy is needed,because the effect of plasmapheresis is transient.

Abstract

For the quantitative analysis of the extraocular muscle changes in Graves' disease,we used B-mode ultrasonography.

113 patients investigated in this study had no signs or symptoms of ophthalmopathy except proptosis.Muscle index was calculated as a sign of extraocular muscle enlargement. Muscle index of Graves' disease was significantly larger than that in controls(6.03 ± 2.83 and 3.10 ± 1.29,respectively).

The muscle index in Graves' patients without clinical signs of exophthalmos was significantly increased when compared to control subjects,although both groups had the same degree of proptosis.The data show a uniform enlargement of the extraocular muscles in Graves' disease.The degree of proptosis is in close proportion to the quantitative change of the orbital soft tissue.

Seven patients with malignant exophthalmos were treated with steroid therapy,supervoltage orbital radiotherapy or plasmapheresis.All patients had moderately severe ophthalmopathy due to Graves' disease.Both steroid therapy and orbital radiation therapy were effective in improving the symptoms of orbital soft tissue involvement and for diplopia.The effect of orbital radiation therapy was insufficient for the amellioration of proptosis in spite of a no significant decrease.The improvement of proptosis was evident only after 3-7 months of the radiotherapy.Plasmapheresis was effective in improving the ulceration of cornea and proptosis,but this was a transient effect.

ACKNOWLEDGEMENTS

Supported in part by a research grant for "Special Disease" of the Japanes Ministry of Health and Welfare.

REFERENCES

Covington,E.E.,Lobes,L.,Sudarsanam,A.1977 Radiation Therapy for exophathalmos:report of seven cases.Radiology 122:797

Donaldson S.S.?Bagshaw M.A.,Kriss,J.P. Supervoltage orbital radiotherapy for Graves' ophthalmopathy.J Clin Endocrinol Metab 37:276

Manley,S.W.,Bourke,J.R.,Hawker,R.W. 1974.The thyrotrophin receptor in guinea-pig thyroid homogenate:General properties J Endocr 61:419

Smith,B.R.,Hall,R.1974.Thyroid-stimulating immunoglobulins in Graves' disease.Lancet ii:427

Teng,C.S.,Crombie,A.L.,Hall,R.,Ross,W.M. 1980 An evaluation of supervoltage orbital irradiation for Graves' ophthalmopathy.Clinical Endocrinology 13:545

Uller,R.P.,Van Herle,A.J. 1978 Effect of therapy on serum thyroglobulin levels in patients with Graves' disease.J Clin Endocrinol Metab 46:747

Van Herle,A.J.,Uller,R.P.,Matthews,N.L.,Brown,J. 1973 Radioimmunoassay for measurement of thyroglobulin in human serum, J Clin Invest 52:1320

Werner,S.C. 1977 Modification of the classification of the eye changes of Graves' disease:Recomendation of the Ad Hoc Comittee of the American Thyroid Association.J Clin Endocrinol Metab 44:203

Winand,R.I. 1968 Increased urinary excretion of acidic mucupolysaccharides in exophthalmos.J Clin Invest 47:2663
Yamamoto,K.,Itoh,K.Yoshida,S.,Saito,K.,Sakamoto,Y.,Matsuda, A.,Saito,T.,Kuzuya,T. 1979 A quantitative analysis of orbital soft tissue in Graves' disease based on B-mode ultrasonography.Endocrinol Japan 26:255

New Concepts in Thyroid Disease, pages 207–223

ON THE THYROTROPIC ACTIVITY OF HUMAN CHORIONIC GONADOTROPIN: ITS ROLE AS THE THYROID STIMULATOR OF TROPHOBLASTIC ORIGIN[1]

Syed M. Amir, Ph.D. and Sidney H. Ingbar, M.D.

Thorndike Laboratory, Beth Israel Hospital

and Harvard Medical School, Boston, MA 02215

For at least twenty years, it has been recognized that thyroid hyperfunction, sometimes severe and occasionally associated with frank thyrotoxicosis, is a common occurrence in patients with trophoblastic tumors (Dowling _et al_. 1960; Odell _et al_. 1963; Cohen _et al_. 1970; Galton _et al_. 1971; Hershman 1972). This is clearly due to the elaboration of a circulating thyroid stimulator by the tumor. This follows from the fact that, as judged from the McKenzie mouse assay (McKenzie 1958), a stimulator is present in the blood of such patients; it disappears from the blood promptly after removal of the tumor, and this is associated with a rapid alleviation of thyroid hyperfunction (Galton _et al_ 1971). The stimulator is certainly not a form of thyrotropin (TSH), similar to that secreted by the pituitary, since it is not detected in the TSH radioimmunoassay (RIA) and since the time course of its action in the mouse assay system is much longer than that of pituitary TSH. Rather, the precise nature of the thyroid stimulator of trophoblastic origin has been a matter of some controversy for years, one view proposing that it is human chorionic gonadotropin (hCG) _per se_, and the other, to which the present authors subscribe, suggesting that it is not.

The present review will consider evidence to this point as well as information concerning certain other thyroid stimulators of presumed placental origin.

[1] Supported by Research Grants CA-31216 and AM-18416, from the National Institutes of Health, Bethesda, MD.

HUMAN CHORIONIC THYROTROPIN AND MOLAR TSH

Only a few years ago, it seemed that the search for placental thyroid stimulators had finally culminated in the successful isolation and partial characterization of two hitherto unrecognized thyroid-stimulating factors (Hennen et al. 1969; Hershman et al. 1970; Hershman, Starnes 1971; Tojo et al. 1973). At this time, however, the significance of these earlier findings appears greatly in doubt, as will be discussed below.

One of the thyroid stimulators whose isolation was initially claimed was extracted from normal placenta and was termed human chorionic TSH (hCT) (Hershman et al. 1970; Hershman, Starnes 1971). Its thyrotropic activity was detected by means of the McKenzie mouse assay system. During chromatography on a Sephadex G-100 column, bioactivity ascribed to hCT eluted at the same position as bovine TSH (bTSH) did, suggesting a similarity in their molecular weights. Material designated as hCT did not cross-react in the RIA for human TSH (hTSH), but did appear to cross-react completely in the RIA for bTSH. In the mouse assay system, hCT had a short duration of action, similar to that of TSH and quite different from the much longer action of the stimulatory material found in the blood of patients with molar pregnancy. Apparent confirmation of these findings was reported by Hennen and co-workers, who extracted and partially purified from normal human placenta a factor that was highly active in an in vivo chick assay for TSH, as well as in the McKenzie mouse assay; the material failed to cross-react in the RIA for hTSH, but did so in the assay for bTSH (Hennen et al. 1969).

Further studies on hCT were reported by Tojo et al. (1973), who extracted it from normal placenta and tested its bioactivity by measuring its ability to increase the radioactive iodine uptake in guinea pig thyroids. They also determined its chemical composition and then developed a specific RIA for its measurement in serum from patients with normal or molar pregnancy. In the RIA for hCT, neither hTSH nor hCG cross-reacted. They claimed that hCT was distinct from hCG in chemical composition, that its serum concentration was much higher in molar than in normal pregnancy, and that its concentration in serum rapidly declined after delivery or removal of

the mole.

Following these early studies, nothing related to hCT was reported until a few years ago, when Harada and Hershman (1978) re-examined the hCT content of normal human placentas. This time, they were unable to obtain a significant recovery of bioactive material in any of their placental extracts, prompting them to suggest that their previous conclusions concerning hCT were invalid and probably had resulted from an inadvertent contamination of their material with bovine TSH. If this was indeed the case, then we are left with the difficulty of reconciling their conclusions with the rather substantial amounts of data on hCT that have been reported independently from other laboratories (Hennen et al. 1969; Tojo et al. 1973). Such reconciliation is not yet possible.

The second putative thyrotropic factor identified in these early studies was extracted from hydatidiform mole and was also identified by its activity in the mouse bioassay system, wherein its stimulatory activity was prolonged (Hershman et al. 1970; Hershman, Higgins 1971). As judged from its behavior during chromatography on a Sephadex G-100 column, its molecular weight appeared to be 60,000-70,000, similar to that of albumin. Unlike hCT, so-called molar TSH (mTSH) did not cross-react in the RIA for either hTSH or bTSH. Apparently, nothing further has been written about mTSH, probably because of a growing interest in the the possibility that mTSH might be the same as hCG.

HCG AS A THYROID STIMULATOR

For approximately a decade, interest has focussed on the possibility that hCG per se is a thyroid stimulator and might be the abnormal thyroid stimulator associated with trophoblastic tumors. The evidence to this point is complex and contradictory, and will be the substance of the remainder of this review. At the outset, it seems important to suggest that this evidence be considered in terms of current concepts of the mode of action of trophic peptide hormones upon their target tissues. These predicate that the action of trophic hormones is initiated by their binding to specific receptors in the target endocrine tissue. Specific binding is followed by biochemical responses which include an activation of adenylate cyclase; the resulting increase in cellular cyclic AMP concentration then initiates a sequence of biochemical sequelae that together comprise much of the over-all reponse to the trophic hormone. Although these aspects of hormone action are most often demonstrated *in vitro*, the ultimate proof of the activity of a putative stimulator rests upon its ability to enhance the activity of its target organ *in vivo*. The controversy concerning the thyroid-stimulating activity of hCG will be examined in this light.

hCG is a Stimulator of the Mouse Thyroid

There is no question that hCG *per se* is capable of stimulating the mouse thyroid gland. This conclusion rests upon a large body of evidence.

The fact that preparations of hCG, like TSH, are capable of stimulating the release of iodine from mouse thyroid in the McKenzie assay system was first unequivocally demonstrated by Burger, who was seeking evidence for the presence of TSH in urine (Burger 1967a; Burger 1967b). Although both crude and purified hCG preparations were active in the mouse assay, Burger attributed this activity to the presence of a contaminating hormone, possibly TSH, in the hCG preparations tested.

Similar findings were later reported by Winand *et al.* (1969), who also tested hCG in the McKenzie mouse assay, but unlike Burger, found that only crude preparations were active. Stimulatory activity of hCG preparations in the mouse assay system was also noted by Uchimura and coworkers (1975).

Prompted by these findings, and in an attempt to clarify the nature of the thyroid stimulator of molar pregnancy, more extensive studies of the thyrotropic activity of hCG were undertaken by several workers. In the studies of Nisula and Ketelslegers (1974), both crude and highly purified preparations of hCG were tested in the mouse bioassay and were found capable of stimulating the thyroid. Furthermore, the gonadotropic and thyrotropic activities were lost when hCG was dissociated into subunits, but were restored when the two subunits were recombined, suggesting that the factor active in the mouse assay was hCG itself.

In a similar study, Kenimer _et al_. (1975) isolated hCG from hydatidiform mole, subjected it to fractionation procedures and studied the relationship between thyrotropic activity, as judged from the mouse assay, and hCG content, as measured by RIA. The authors estimated that each unit of hCG contains 0.5 uU of TSH activity. From their findings, the authors concluded that hCG and mTSH were the same, and that hCG is, therefore, the thyroid stimulator of molar pregnancy.

As we have discussed in detail elsewhere (Amir _et al_. 1980), there are aspects of these data that do not accord with the conclusion that hCG _per se_ is the only stimulator of mouse thyroid present in crude hCG preparations. First, and most important, in the report of Kenimer _et al_. cited above, sequential fractionation of crude hCG yielded fractions progressively enriched in thyrotropic activity, but without concurrent enrichment in hCG. Further, among a number of highly and partially purified preparations of hCG, very wide differences were noted in ratios of mouse thyroid stimulatory activity to hCG content, measured by either RIA or by bioassay.

Data from our own laboratory have provided evidence at a biochemical level that hCG is capable of stimulating the mouse thyroid with a reasonable degree of potency (Amir _et al_. 1982a). Preparations of highly purified, ^{125}I-labeled hCG (^{125}I-hCG) display specific and saturable binding to mouse thyroid membranes _in vitro_, and in studies of mouse thyroids incubated _in vitro_, pure hCG could be shown to stimulate the release of both cyclic AMP and thyroxine (T_4) into the medium.

Thus, by all the criteria described above, hCG can be considered a significant stimulator of the mouse thyroid gland, but as judged from the data of Kenimer _et al_. (1975), it is possible that some other component in crude hCG is also capable of stimulating the mouse thyroid.

Possible Role of Species Variations

The certainty that hCG _per se_ is a stimulator of the

mouse thyroid does not necessarily dictate, however, that it is also a significantly potent stimulator of the human thyroid gland, since many instances of species-related variations in the response of the thyroid to various stimulators can be cited. Thus, as demonstrated by Odell and coworkers (1963), the chick thyroid, unlike that of the mouse, is insensitive to hCG. Similarly, in our own studies, preparations of ^{125}I-hCG bind little, if at all, to human thyroid membranes, but bind very well to mouse thyroid membranes (Amir *et al*. 1982a).

Equally striking species-dependent differences are evident in the case of the thyroid-stimulating immunoglobulins (IgG) of Graves' disease. Those Graves'-IgG capable of stimulating the mouse thyroid have been defined as having long-acting thyroid stimulatory activity (LATS), since their action in the mouse is more prolonged than that of TSH. It has long been known, however, that preparations of Graves' -IgG active in the LATS assay are inactive in the chick assay (Lepp, Oliver 1967). Similarly, certain preparations active in the LATS assay fail to enhance cyclic AMP concentration in guinea pig and dog thyroid *in vitro* (Zakarija, McKenzie 1978). Also, some preparations have been shown to be active both in the LATS assay and *in vitro* human assays, while others have been found to be active only in the human assay (Zakarija, McKenzie 1978; Adams, Kennedy 1971). More importantly, assays for bioactive Graves'-IgG display a much higher frequency of positivity and a closer correlation with clinical state than assays employing the mouse do (McKenzie, Zakarija 1976).

It has been debated whether findings such as those noted above reflect absolute insensitivity of the thyroids of certain species to particular stimulators or merely wide variations in sensitivity, ranging from the highly sensitive to the highly insensitive. Nonetheless, from the standpoint of the present discussion, this difference is not critical, since the question under consideration is whether hCG is a sufficiently potent stimulator of human thyroid to qualify as the agent responsible for thyroid hyperfunction in patients with trophoblastic tumors.

hCG as Human Thyroid Stimulator: *In Vitro* Studies.

Evidence that hCG is a human thyroid stimulator. Those

who advocate the view that hCG is a human thyroid stimulator of significant potency have brought forward the results of both _in vitro_ studies and observations in patients in support of this postulate. Among the _in vitro_ studies are some related to the binding of hCG to human thyroid membranes and one study of the ability of hCG to activate adenylate cyclase cyclase therein.

Binding of hCG to human thyroid membranes has been studied in two ways, by examining the direct binding of ^{125}I-hCG to membrane preparations and by demonstrating the ability of hCG to inhibit the binding of ^{125}I-labeled bTSH (^{125}I-bTSH). Direct binding of ^{125}I-labeled preparations of hCG to human thyroid membranes was first studied by Azukizawa _et al_. (1977). These authors labeled crude hCG with ^{125}I and fractionated it by chromatography on Ultrogel AcA44 resin. The fraction found to be most active in a receptor assay for hCG, using the rat testis, was then incubated with human thyroid membranes, and displayed approximately 3% specific binding. However, when highly purified hCG was ^{125}I-labeled, its specific binding to human thyroid membranes was less than 1%. This discrepancy raises the possibility that much of the binding which these authors found with fractionated crude hCG was due to some factor other than intact hCG itself.

A more detailed study of this subject was conducted by Carayon _et al_. (1980). They "receptor-purified" a preparation of radiolabeled purified hCG by means of human thyroid membranes. Nonetheless, maximum binding of the resulting tracer to increasing quantities of human thyroid membranes was only 2%. Further, the preparation of ^{125}I-hCG receptor-purified with human thyroid membranes displayed a greater binding to rat testis membranes than the original preparation of ^{125}I-hCG did. This suggests that the original hCG preparation was not entirely homogeneous, and it raises the question of whether it was a contaminant or hCG _per se_ that was binding to the thyroid.

Other studies, apart from our own, have examined the ability of crude and purified hCG to inhibit the binding of ^{125}I-bTSH to human thyroid membranes. (Davies _et al_. [1979] have used this approach to study the binding of hCG to porcine thyroid membranes, but for reasons cited above related to the problem of species specificity, these findings are not necessarily applicable to the present question.) Pekonen and Weintraub (1980) have compared the TSH-displacing activity of crude and pure hCG in the human thyroid membrane and have concluded that the conditions of study greatly influence the relative potencies of the two. Thus, when the incubation was performed at low temperature (4° C) and in low salt (20 mM Tris) medium, the cross-reactivities of crude and purified hCG with TSH were 90% and less than 0.01%, respectively, on a molar basis. However, when tested under what was described as "near physiological" conditions (37° C, 50 mM NaCl), the activities of crude and purified hCG were greatly reduced relative to that of TSH and were equal. Under these conditions, purified hCG at the highest concentration employed (2.8×10^{-6}M; 1,489 IU/ml), inhibited ^{125}I-bTSH binding to human human thyroid membrane by only 10%. The authors estimated a 0.003-0.005% cross-reactivity of hCG in their receptor assay. Despite this, they favored the view that hCG has intrinsic TSH-like activity. In earlier studies, Silverberg et al. (1978) had demonstrated that preparations of crude hCG inhibited the binding of ^{125}I-bTSH to human thyroid membranes when studied at 37° C in the presence of 50 mM NaCl. However, pure hCG was not tested; as a consequence, the nature of the inhibitory material in the preparations they used cannot be ascertained.

Two groups, apart from our own, have studied the ability of hCG to stimulate adenylate cyclase in human thyroid membranes or slices. The question was first approached by Silverberg et al. (1978). Crude hCG produced a pronounced increase in cAMP concentration in slices of human thyroid, but two problems complicate the interpretation of these findings. First, purified hCG was not tested. Second, the preparation of crude hCG that they employed contained benzyl alcohol and phenol. Both of these agents are capable of producing a strong stimulation of adenylate cyclase in human thyroid membranes (Amir et al. 1981a).

Carayon et al. (1980), in the study cited earlier, examined the ability of pure hCG to stimulate adenylate cyclase in human thyroid membranes. A very slight stimulatory response was noted, but the maximum increase achieved by the most effective concentration was approximately 15% While it remains uncertain whether this low degree of stimulation is biologically meaningful, the problem is further complicated by the fact that the maximum response to TSH, an indication of the sensitivity of the system, was not described. An estimate of the TSH-like potency of pure hCG was was presented (0.27 uU/IU hCG), but this was based upon a comparison of minimum concentrations required to enhance adenylate cyclase activity. This rather imprecise means of estimating relative potencies may have been adopted because of the very low level of hCG activity seen. Further, it should be noted that in these experiments, similar increases in enzyme activity were produced by equal weights of pure hCG and crude hCG, although the latter contained only one-one-fourth the hCG bioactivity, a finding hardly compatible with the claim that hCG itself was the active agent.

Evidence that hCG is not a significant human thyroid stimulator. The possibility that hCG is a sufficiently potent stimulator of the human thyroid to account for the thyroid hyperfunction associated with trophoblastic tumors is a question that has attracted the interest and activity of our laboratory for quite some time. Our studies have persuaded us that it is not.

Our early studies to this point were performed using bovine thyroid tissue (Amir *et al*. 1977), before we had ourselves recognized the possible role of species-related variations in response. Although the data provided essentially no support for a significant stimulatory activity of hCG *per se*, we must now dismiss the relevance of these findings to the present question, as we have in the case of the studies of Davies *et al*. (1979) with porcine thyroid tissue, cited above. More recently, however, we have examined the question in preparations of human thyroid membranes and human thyroid slices (Amir *et al*. 1980; Uchimura *et al*. 1982). First, as regards the direct binding of ^{125}I-hCG to human thyroid membranes, we too found this to be negligible (0.5%) in membrane preparations which bound a high proportion of ^{125}I-bTSH. This was true even under conditions of temperature (4° C) and salt concentration (20 mM Tris, no NaCl) which favor binding of hCG relative to that of TSH, as judged from the ability of hCG to inhibit TSH binding. For this reason, we employed the ability of hCG preparations to inhibit the binding of ^{125}I-bTSH as an index of their own ability to bind to human thyroid membranes (Amir *et al*. 1980). In these studies, a consistent finding has been that, when compared on the basis of equivalent gonadotropic activity, crude hCG was far more potent (10-40 fold) than pure hCG. This high potency ratio was observed in studies carried out at 4° C in the absence of

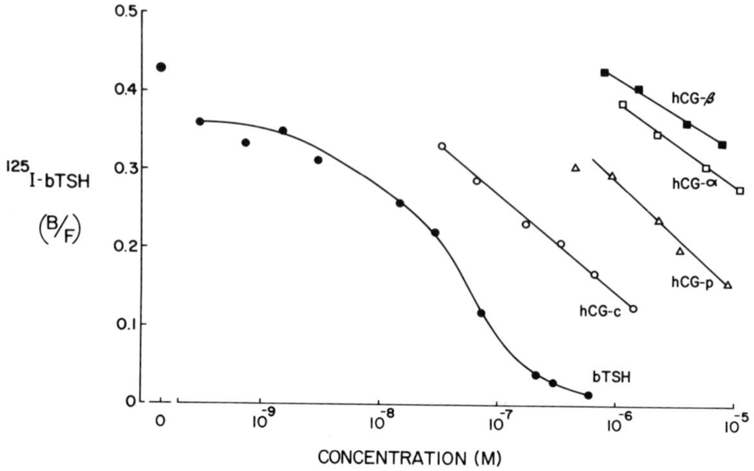

Fig. 1. Inhibition of ^{125}I-bTSH binding to human thyroid membranes by unlabeled bTSH, crude hCG (hCG-c), purified hCG (hCG-p) and hCG-subunits (4°C, 20 mM Tris pH 7.45) (From Amir et al., 1980, J Clin Endocrinol Metab 51:51).

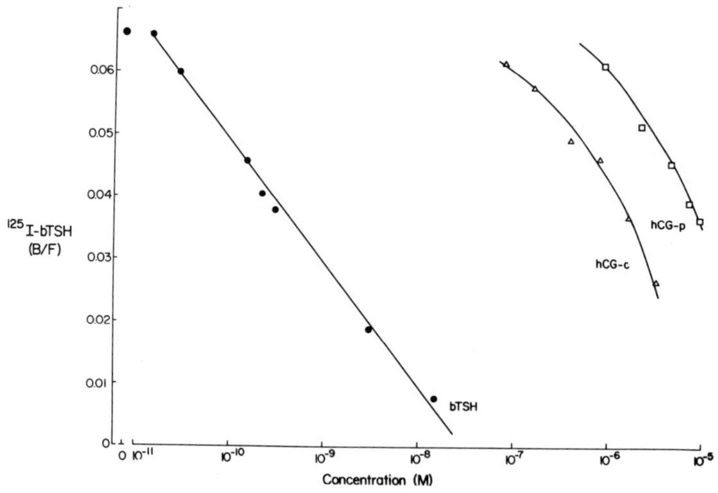

Fig. 2. Inhibition of ^{125}I-bTSH binding to human thyroid membranes by unlabeled bTSH, hCG-c and hCG-p (37°C, 50 mM NaCl) (From Amir et al., 1980, J Clin Endocrinol Metab 51:51).

salt (Figure 1), but a greater potency of crude hCG (4-fold) was also evident under "physiological" conditions (37° C and 50 mM NaCl) (Figure 2). These findings suggest that some factor(s) other than intact hCG itself may be largely responsible for the inhibition of TSH binding seen with crude preparations. Possibilities for such factors include desialylated hCG, which we have shown to have increased binding affinity for human thyroid membranes (Amir et al. 1981b), or hCG lacking its carboxy-terminal amino acid, which has enhanced potency in stimulating thyroid adenylate cyclase (Carayon et al. 1981).

In two separate studies, we have also examined the ability of preparations of hCG to stimulate adenylate cyclase or increase cyclic AMP concentration in human thyroid tissue In the first (Amir et al. 1980), crude thyroid membrane preparations were employed. Although the preparations were quite responsive to bTSH, they failed to respond to either crude or pure hCG. This was true even at concentrations of hCG (2,000-40,000 IU/ml) that should have yielded activity comparable to that of TSH, had the hCG displayed a TSH-like activity with a potency equal to that ascribed to it by Kenimer et al. (1975) on the basis of its activity in the mouse assay (Figure 3). Further to the point, crude hCG proved capable of inhibiting the adenylate cyclase response to bTSH, but pure hCG did not.

The second study was carried out using human thyroid slices, a system more sensitive to stimulators than the crude membrane preparation is. Here, concentrations of pure hCG as high as 4,000 IU/ml (bioassay) failed to increase cyclic AMP concentration, though crude hCG over a concentration range of 3,000-5,000 IU/ml produced a significant stimulation (Uchimura et al. 1982) (Figure 4). As in the membrane system, crude hCG was capable of inhibiting the stimulatory response to bTSH in the slices, while purified hCG, in similar amounts that contained approximately 5-times the hCG bioactivity, was not.

Thus, as can be seen from the results of our studies, there is a distinct parallelism between the studies of the binding of crude vs pure hCG to human thyroid membranes and their ability to influence adenylate cyclase activity, the evidence indicating that crude hCG interacts with the human thyroid to a far greater extent than pure hCG does.

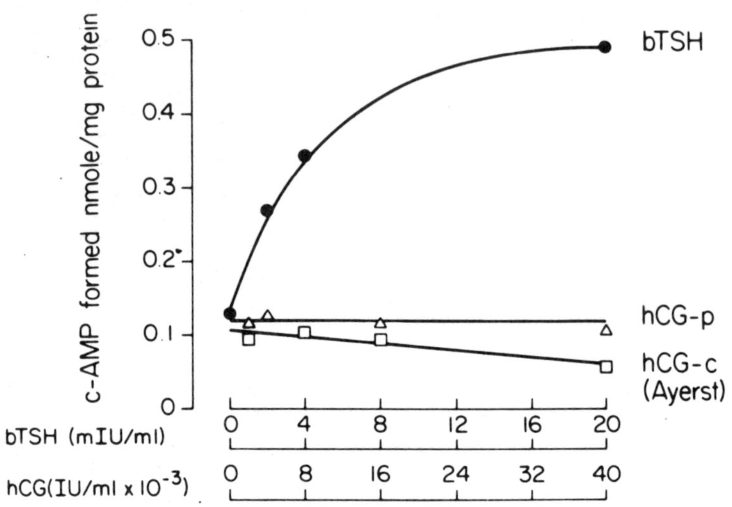

Fig. 3. Effect of bTSH, hCG-c and hCG-p on adenylate cyclase activation in human thyroid membranes (From Amir _et al_., 1980, J Clin Endocrinol Metab 51:51).

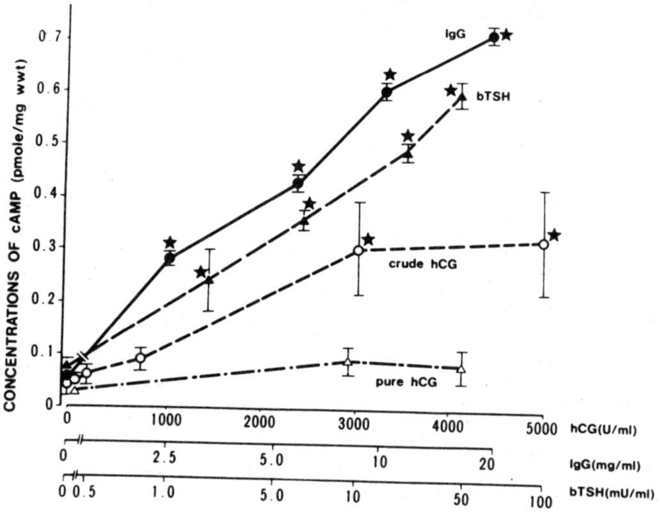

Fig. 4. Effect of bTSH, hCG-c and hCG-p on cyclic AMP accumulation in human thyroid slices (From Uchimura _et_ al., 1982, J Clin Endocrinol Metab 55:347).

hCG as a Human Thyroid Stimulator: *In Vivo* Studies.

Evidently, only one study has addressed the question of whether hCG can stimulate the human thyroid *in vivo*. Sowers *et al*. (1978) have administered very large amounts (100,000–150,000 IU) of a crude hCG preparation to 8 euthyroid volunteers whose thyroids had been pre-labeled with ^{125}I. A highly sensitive technique for detecting stimulation of thyroid iodine release (Nicoloff, 1970) was employed. Only a slight increase in thyroid iodine release was noted, and serum T_4, T_3, and TSH concentraations were unchanged over the ensuing 48 hours. This minimal evidence of thyroid stimulation was obtained despite the fact that serum hCG concentrations as high as 2532 IU/ml were achieved. Had the hCG had a TSH bioactivity in man equivalent to its estimated activity in the mouse (Kenimer *et al*. 1975), a serum TSH concentration of 12-16 uU/ml would have been expected, and this should have been sufficient to produce a detectable stimulation by the techniques employed. Even if a clear stimulation had been seen, conclusions concerning the role of hCG *per se* would have been clouded, since crude, rather than pure, hCG was administered, and since the preparation contained phenol and benzyl alcohol, both known to be *in vitro* thyroid stimulators. (Amir *et al*. 1981a).

A less direct approach to the question of whether hCG has significant stimulatory activity in man is represented by efforts to correlate the level of thyroid function in patients with trophoblastic tumors with their serum hCG levels. However, such studies have recently undergone extensive review, in conjunction with a report of our own findings in this respect. Therefore, a review of all the findings cannot be undertaken here. In general, however, these correlative studies studies provide no definitive evidence, in our view, to support the hypothesis that hCG itself is the thyroid stimulator of molar pregnancy (Amir *et al*.1982b).

CONCLUSIONS

We believe that the weight of the evidence cited above strongly favors the suggestion that intact hCG, though clearly a significant stimulator of the mouse thyroid, has little or no thyroid stimulatory activity in man. Therefore, it is unlikely to be the abnormal thyroid stimulator that that is responsible for thyroid hyperfunction in patients with trophoblastic tumors. Nonetheless, there is, in preparations of crude hCG one or more factors that are capable of stimulating the human thyroid gland, at least as judged from responses observed in human thyroid slices in vitro. The nature of such factors remains conjectural, however. They are unlikely to be desialylated forms of hCG; though these can bind to human thyroid membranes with reasonable affinity, we have been unable to demonstrate that they have any stimulatory action therein. Conceivably, the stimulatory factors in crude hCG could be forms of hCG, with modified caboxy-terminal regions, since such preparations have been shown to have increased potency in stimulating adenylate cyclase in human thyroid tissue (Carayon et al. 1981). It is uncertain, however, whether the latter variants of hCG are indeed present in crude hCG preparations or are formed from hCG in vivo, either during normal pregnancy or in patients with trophoblastic tumors.

The recent finding of a thyroid-stimulating protein that is extractable from bovine placenta and is distinct from bTSH and hCG revives the concept of a chorionic thyrotropin (Avivi et al. 1982). The bovine material has a much higher molecular weight (94,000 dalton) than either human or bovine TSH, does not cross-react in the RIA for bTSH, and displays no gonadotropic activity in vitro. In the light of this, and in view of the earlier work of Hennen et al. (1969) and Tojo et al. (1973), it may be premature to dismiss the possible existence of a human chorionic thyrotropin that is distinct from hCG. The question clearly warrants further exploration.

REFERENCES

Adams A, Kennedy TH (1971). Evidence to suggest that LATS protector stimulates the human thyroid gland. J Clin Endocrinol Metab 33:47.

Amir SM, Uchimura H, Ingbar, SH (1977). Interactions of bovine thyrotropin with bovine thyroid membranes. J Clin Endocrinol Metab 45:280.

Amir SM, Sullivan RC, Ingbar SH (1980). In vitro responses to crude and purified hCG in human thyroid membranes. J J Clin Endocrinol Metab 51:51.

Amir SM, Mulrow NJ, Ingbar SH (1981a). Phenol, a potent

stimulator of adenylate cyclase in human thyroid membranes. Endocr Res Commun 8:83.

Amir SM, Sullivan RC, Ingbar SH (1981b). The effect of desialylation on the in vitro interaction of human chorionic gonadotropin with human thyroid membranes. Endocrinology 109:1203.

Amir SM, Kane P, Osathanondh R (1982a). Divergent responses by human and mouse thyroids to human chorionic gonadotropin (hCG) in vitro. Program of the 64th Annual Meeting of the Endocrine Society, Abstract No. 1222.

Amir SM, Osathanondh R, Berkowitz RS, Goldstein DD, Ingbar SH (1982b). Human chorionic gonadotropin and thyroid function in patients with hydatidiform mole. Am J Obstet Gynecol (submitted for publication).

Avivi A, Schreiber AB, Shemesh M (1982). Isolation and characterization of a 94,000-dalton protein with thyrotropic activity from early bovine placenta. J Biol Chem 257:11384.

Azukizawa M, Kurtzman G, Pekary AE, Hershman JM (1977). Comparison of the binding characteristics of bovine thyrotropin and human chorionic gonadotropin to thyroid plasma membranes. Endocrinology 101:1880.

Burger A (1967a). Studies on a thyroid-stimulating factor in urinary chorionic gonadotropin preparations. Acta Endocrinol (Kbh) 55:587.

Burger A (1967b). Further studies on a thyroid-stimulating factor in crude chorionic gonadotropin preparations and in urine. Acta Endocrinol (Kbh) 55:600.

Carayon P, Lefort G, Nisula B (1980). Interaction of human chorionic gonadotropin and human luteinizing hormone with human thyroid membranes. Endocrinology 106:1907.

Carayon P, Amr S, Nisula B. Lissitzky S (1981). Effects of carboxypeptidase digestion of the human chorionic gonadotropin molecule on its thyrotropic activity. Endocrinology 108:1891.

Cohen JD, Utiger RD (1970). Metastatic choriocarcinoma associated with hyperthyroidism. J Clin Endocrinol Metab 30:423.

Davies TF, Taliadouros GS, Catt KJ, Nisula BC (1979). Assessment of urinary thyrotropin-competing activity in choriocarcinoma and thyroid disease: Further evidence for human chorionic gonadotropin interacting at the thyroid membrane. J Clin Endocrinol Metab 49:353.

Dowling JT, Ingbar SH, Freinkel N (1960). Iodine metabolism in hydatidiform mole and choriocarcinoma. J Clin Endocrinol Metab 21:1.

Galton VA, Ingbar SH, Jiminez-Fonseca J, Hershman JM (1971) Alterations in thyroid hormone economy in patients with hydatidiform mole. J Clin Invest 50:1345.
Harada A, Hershman JM (1978). Extraction of human chorionic thyrotropin (hCT) from term placentas: Failure to recover thyrotropic activity. J Clin Endocrinol Met 47:681.
Hennen G, Pierce JG, Freychet P (1969). Human chorionic thyrotropin: Further characterization and study of its secretion during pregnancy. J Clin Endocrinol Metab 29: 581.
Hershman JM, Higgins HP, Starnes WR (1970). Differences between thyroid stimulator in hydatidiform mole and human chorionic thyrotropin. Metabolism 19:735.
Hershman JM, Higgins HP (1971). Hydatidiform mole: A cause of clinical hyperthyroidism. N Engl J Med 284:573.
Hershman JM, Starnes WR (1971). Placental content and characterisation of human chorionic thyrotropin. J Clin Endocrinol Metab 32:52.
Hershman JM (1972). Hyperthyroidism induced by trophoblastic thyrotropin. Mayo Clin Proc 47:913.
Kenimer JG, Hershman JM, Higgins HP (1975). The thyrotropin in hydatidiform moles is human chorionic gonadotropin. J Clin Endocrinol Metab 40:482.
Lepp A, Oliver L (1967). Failure of long-acting thyroid stimulator globulin (LATS) and serum to stimulate thyroid function in the chick. Endocrinology 80:369.
McKenzie JM (1958). The bioassay of thyrotropin in serum. Endocrinology 63:372.
McKenzie JM, Zakarija M (1976). A reconsideration of a thyroid-stimulating immunoglobulin as the cause of hyperthyroidism in Graves'disease. J Clin Endocrinol Metab 42:778.
Nicoloff JT (1970). A new method for the measurement of thyroidal iodine release in man. J Clin Invest 49:1912.
Nisula BC, Ketelslegers JM (1974). Thyroid-stimulating activity and chorionic gonadotropin. J Clin Invest 54: 494.
Odell WD, Bates RW, Rivlin RS, Lipsett MB, Hertz R (1963). Increased thyroid function without clinical hyperthyroidism in patients with choriocarcinoma. J Clin Endocrinol Metab 23:658.
Pekonen F, Weintraub BD (1980). Interactions of crude and pure chorionic gonadotropin with the thyrotropin receptor. J Clin Endocrinol Metab 50:28.
Silverberg J, O'Donnell J, Sugenaya A, Row VV and Volpe R

(1978). Effects of human chorionic gonadotropin on human thyroid tissue in vitro. J Clin Endocrinol Metab 46:420.
Sowers JR, Hershman JM, Carlson HE, Pekary AE (1978). Effect of human chorionic gonadotropin on thyroid function in euthyroid men. J Clin Endocrinol Metab 47:898.
Tojo S, Kanazawa S, Nakamura A, Kitagaki S, Mochizuku M (1973). Human chorionic TSH (hCTSH, hCT) during normal or molar pregnancy. Endocrinol Japan 20:505.
Uchimura H, Nagataki S, Tabuchi T. Mizumo M, Ito K (1975). The thyroid-stimulating activity of highly purified preparations of human chorionic gonadotropin, Proceeding of the Seventh International Thyroid Conference, Boston, Excerpta Medica International Congress Series, No. 378, p.37.
Uchimura H, Nagataki S, Ito K, Amir SM, Ingbar SH (1982). Inhibition of the adenylate cyclase response to thyroid-stimulating immunoglobulin G by crude and asialo-human chorionic gonadotropin. J Clin Endocrinol Metab 55:347.
Winand R, Bates R, Becker CE, Rosen SW (1969). Unusual thyroid-stimulating activity in the plasma of a man with choriocarcinoma. J Clin Endocrinol Metab 29:1369.

Index

PROGRESS IN CLINICAL AND BIOLOGICAL RESEARCH

Series Editors
Nathan Back
George J. Brewer
Vincent P. Eijsvoogel
Robert Grover
Kurt Hirschhorn
Seymour S. Kety
Sidney Udenfriend
Jonathan W. Uhr

Vol 1: **Erythrocyte Structure and Function,** George J. Brewer, *Editor*

Vol 2: **Preventability of Perinatal Injury,** Karlis Adamsons, Howard A. Fox, *Editors*

Vol 3: **Infections of the Fetus and the Newborn Infant,** Saul Krugman, Anne A. Gershon, *Editors*

Vol 4: **Conflicts in Childhood Cancer: An Evaluation of Current Management,** Lucius F. Sinks, John O. Godden, *Editors*

Vol 5: **Trace Components of Plasma: Isolation and Clinical Significance,** G.A. Jamieson, T.J. Greenwalt, *Editors*

Vol 6: **Prostatic Disease,** H. Marberger, H. Haschek, H.K.A. Schirmer, J.A.C. Colston, E. Witkin, *Editors*

Vol 7: **Blood Pressure, Edema and Proteinuria in Pregnancy,** Emanuel A. Friedman, *Editor*

Vol 8: **Cell Surface Receptors,** Garth L. Nicolson, Michael A. Raftery, Martin Rodbell, C. Fred Fox, *Editors*

Vol 9: **Membranes and Neoplasia: New Approaches and Strategies,** Vincent T. Marchesi, *Editor*

Vol 10: **Diabetes and Other Endocrine Disorders During Pregnancy and in the Newborn,** Maria I. New, Robert H. Fiser, *Editors*

Vol 11: **Clinical Uses of Frozen-Thawed Red Blood Cells,** John A. Griep, *Editor*

Vol 12: **Breast Cancer,** Albert C.W. Montague, Geary L. Stonesifer, Jr., Edward F. Lewison, *Editors*

Vol 13: **The Granulocyte: Function and Clinical Utilization,** Tibor J. Greenwalt, G.A. Jamieson, *Editors*

Vol 14: **Zinc Metabolism: Current Aspects in Health and Disease,** George J. Brewer, Ananda S. Prasad, *Editors*

Vol 15: **Cellular Neurobiology,** Zach Hall, Regis Kelly, C. Fred Fox, *Editors*

Vol 16: **HLA and Malignancy,** Gerald P. Murphy, *Editor*

Vol 17: **Cell Shape and Surface Architecture,** Jean Paul Revel, Ulf Henning, C. Fred Fox, *Editors*

Vol 18: **Tay-Sachs Disease: Screening and Prevention,** Michael M. Kaback, *Editor*

Vol 19: **Blood Substitutes and Plasma Expanders,** G.A. Jamieson, T.J. Greenwalt, *Editors*

Vol 20: **Erythrocyte Membranes: Recent Clinical and Experimental Advances,** Walter C. Kruckeberg, John W. Eaton, George J. Brewer, *Editors*

Vol 21: **The Red Cell,** George J. Brewer, *Editor*

Volume 22: **Molecular Aspects of Membrane Transport,** Dale Oxender, C. Fred Fox, *Editors*

Vol 23: **Cell Surface Carbohydrates and Biological Recognition,** Vincent T. Marchesi, Victor Ginsburg, Phillips W. Robbins, C. Fred Fox, *Editors*

Vol 24: **Twin Research, Proceedings of the Second International Congress on Twin Studies,** Walter E. Nance, *Editor* Published in 3 volumes: Part A: **Psychology and Methodology** Part B: **Biology and Epidemiology** Part C: **Clinical Studies**

Vol 25: **Recent Advances in Clinical Oncology,** Tapan A. Hazra, Michael C. Beachley, *Editors*

Vol 26: **Origin and Natural History of Cell Lines,** Claudio Barigozzi, *Editor*

Vol 27: **Membrane Mechanisms of Drugs of Abuse,** Charles W. Sharp, Leo G. Abood, *Editors*

Vol 28: **The Blood Platelet in Transfusion Therapy,** G.A. Jamieson, Tibor J. Greenwalt, *Editors*

Vol 29: **Biomedical Applications of the Horseshoe Crab (Limulidae),** Elias Cohen, *Editor-in-Chief*

Vol 30: **Normal and Abnormal Red Cell Membranes,** Samuel E. Lux, Vincent T. Marchesi, C. Fred Fox, *Editors*

Vol 31: **Transmembrane Signaling,** Mark Bitensky, R. John Collier, Donald F. Steiner, C. Fred Fox, *Editors*

Vol 32: **Genetic Analysis of Common Diseases: Applications to Predictive Factors in Coronary Disease,** Charles F. Sing, Mark Skolnick, *Editors*

Vol 33: **Prostate Cancer and Hormone Receptors,** Gerald P. Murphy, Avery A. Sandberg, *Editors*

Vol 34: **The Management of Genetic Disorders,** Constantine J. Papadatos, Christos S. Bartsocas, *Editors*

Vol 35: **Antibiotics and Hospitals,** Carlo Grassi, Giuseppe Ostino, *Editors*

Vol 36: **Drug and Chemical Risks to the Fetus, Newborn,** Richard H. Schwarz, Sumner J. Yaffe, *Editors*

Vol 37: **Models for Prostate Cancer,** Gerald P. Murphy, *Editor*

Vol 38: **Ethics, Humanism, and Medicine,** Marc D. Basson, *Editor*

Vol 39: **Neurochemistry and Clinical Neurology,** Leontino Battistin, George Hashim, Abel Lajtha, *Editors*

Vol 40: **Biological Recognition and Assembly,** David S. Eisenberg, James A. Lake, C. Fred Fox, *Editors*

Vol 41: **Tumor Cell Surfaces and Malignancy,** Richard O. Hynes, C. Fred Fox, *Editors*

Vol 42: **Membranes, Receptors, and the Immune Response: 80 Years After Ehrlich's Side Chain Theory,** Edward P. Cohen, Heinz Köhler, *Editors*

Vol 43: **Immunobiology of the Erythrocyte,** S. Gerald Sandler, Jacob Nusbacher, Moses S. Schanfield, *Editors*

Vol 44: **Perinatal Medicine Today,** Bruce K. Young, *Editor*

Vol 45: **Mammalian Genetics and Cancer: The Jackson Laboratory Fiftieth Anniversary Symposium,** Elizabeth S. Russell, *Editor*

Vol 46: **Etiology of Cleft Lip and Cleft Palate,** Michael Melnick, David Bixler, Edward D. Shields, *Editors*

Vol 47: **New Developments With Human and Veterinary Vaccines,** A. Mizrahi, I. Hertman, M.A. Klingberg, A. Kohn, *Editors*

Vol 48: **Cloning of Human Tumor Stem Cells,** Sidney E. Salmon, *Editor*

Vol 49: **Myelin: Chemistry and Biology,** George A. Hashim, *Editor*

Vol 50: **Rights and Responsibilities in Modern Medicine: The Second Volume in a Series on Ethics, Humanism, and Medicine,** Marc D. Basson, *Editor*

Vol 51: **The Function of Red Blood Cells: Erythrocyte Pathobiology,** Donald F. H. Wallach, *Editor*

Vol 52: **Conduction Velocity Distributions: A Population Approach to Electrophysiology of Nerve,** Leslie J. Dorfman, Kenneth L. Cummins, Lary J. Leifer, *Editors*

Vol 53: **Cancer Among Black Populations,** Curtis Mettlin, Gerald P. Murphy, *Editors*

Vol 54: **Connective Tissue Research: Chemistry, Biology, and Physiology,** Zdenek Deyl, Milan Adam, *Editors*

Vol 55: **The Red Cell: Fifth Ann Arbor Conference,** George J. Brewer, *Editor*

Vol 56: **Erythrocyte Membranes 2: Recent Clinical and Experimental Advances,** Walter C. Kruckeberg, John W. Eaton, George J. Brewer, *Editors*

Vol 57: **Progress in Cancer Control,** Curtis Mettlin, Gerald P. Murphy, *Editors*

Vol 58: **The Lymphocyte,** Kenneth W. Sell, William V. Miller, *Editors*

Vol 59: **Eleventh International Congress of Anatomy,** Enrique Acosta Vidrio, *Editor-in-Chief.* Published in 3 volumes: Part A: **Glial and Neuronal Cell Biology,** Sergey Fedoroff, *Editor* Part B: **Advances in the Morphology of Cells and Tissues,** Miguel A. Galina, *Editor* Part C: **Biological Rhythms in Structure and Function,** Heinz von Mayersbach, Lawrence E. Scheving, John E. Pauly, *Editors*

Vol 60: **Advances in Hemoglobin Analysis,** Samir M. Hanash, George J. Brewer, *Editors*

Vol 61: **Nutrition and Child Health: Perspectives for the 1980s,** Reginald C. Tsang, Buford Lee Nichols, Jr., *Editors*

Vol 62: **Pathophysiological Effects of Endotoxins at the Cellular Level,** Jeannine A. Majde, Robert J. Person, *Editors*

Vol 63: **Membrane Transport and Neuroreceptors,** Dale Oxender, Arthur Blume, Ivan Diamond, C. Fred Fox, *Editors*

Vol 64: **Bacteriophage Assembly,** Michael S. DuBow, *Editor*

Vol 65: **Apheresis: Development, Applications, and Collection Procedures,** C. Harold Mielke, Jr., *Editor*

Vol 66: **Control of Cellular Division and Development,** Dennis Cunningham, Eugene Goldwasser, James Watson, C. Fred Fox, *Editors.* Published in 2 volumes.

Vol 67: **Nutrition in the 1980s: Contraints on Our Knowledge,** Nancy Selvey, Philip L. White, *Editors*

Vol 68: **The Role of Peptides and Amino Acids as Neurotransmitters,** J. Barry Lombardini, Alexander D. Kenny, *Editors*

Vol 69: **Twin Research 3, Proceedings of the Third International Congress on Twin Studies,** Ligi Gedda, Paolo Parisi, Walter E. Nance, *Editors.* Published in 3 volumes: Part A: **Twin Biology and Multiple Pregnancy** Part B: **Intelligence, Personality, and Development** Part C: **Epidemiological and Clinical Studies**

Vol 70: **Reproductive Immunology,** Norbert Gleicher, *Editor*

Vol 71: **Psychopharmacology of Clonidine,** Harbans Lal, Stuart Fielding, *Editors*

Vol 72: **Hemophilia and Hemostasis,** Doris Ménaché, D. MacN. Surgenor, Harlan D. Anderson, *Editors*

Vol 73: **Membrane Biophysics: Structure and Function in Epithelia,** Mumtaz A. Dinno, Arthur B. Callahan, *Editors*

Vol 74: **Physiopathology of Endocrine Diseases and Mechanisms of Hormone Action,** Roberto J. Soto, Alejandro De Nicola, Jorge Blaquier, *Editors*

Vol 75: **The Prostatic Cell: Structure and Function,** Gerald P. Murphy, Avery A. Sandberg, James P. Karr, *Editors.* Published in 2 volumes: Part A: **Morphologic, Secretory, and Biochemical Aspects** Part B: **Prolactin, Carcinogenesis, and Clinical Aspects**

Vol 76: **Troubling Problems in Medical Ethics: The Third Volume in a Series on Ethics, Humanism, and Medicine,** Marc D. Basson, Rachel E. Lipson, Doreen L. Ganos, *Editors*

Vol 77: **Nutrition in Health and Disease and International Development: Symposia From the XII International Congress of Nutrition,** Alfred E. Harper, George K. Davis *Editors*

Vol 78: **Female Incontinence,** Norman R. Zinner, Arthur M. Sterling, *Editors*